READY REFERENCE FOR **CRITICAL CARE**
Second Edition

Rhonda M. Strawn, RN, MS, CCRN
Gulfport, Mississippi

Bonnie P. Stewart, RNCS, MS, CCRN
Biloxi, Mississippi

JONES AND BARTLETT PUBLISHERS
Sudbury, Massachusetts

Boston   London   Singapore

Editorial, Sales, and Customer Service Offices
Jones and Bartlett Publishers
40 Tall Pine Drive
Sudbury, MA 01776
508-443-5000
info@jbpub.com
http://www.jbpub.com

Jones and Bartlett Publishers International
Barb House, Barb Mews
London W6 7PA
UK

Copyright © 1997, 1993 Jones and Bartlett Publishers, Inc.

Library of Congress Cataloging-in-Publication Data

Strawn, Rhonda M.
   Ready reference for critical care / Rhonda M. Strawn, Bonnie P.
Stewart. — 2nd ed.
         p.   cm.
   Includes bibliographical references.
   ISBN 978-0-7637-0251-9
   1. Intensive care nursing—Handbooks, manuals, etc.   2. Critical
care medicine—Handbooks, manuals, etc.   I. Stewart, Bonnie P.
II. Title.
   [DNLM: 1. Nursing Care—handbooks.   2. Critical Care—handbooks.
3. Critical Care—Nurses' instruction.   WY 49 S913r 1997]
RT120.I5S77   1997
610.73'61--dc21
DNLM/DLC
for Library of Congress   96-37503
                                                              CIP

Printed in the United States of America
01   00   99   98   97   10   9   8   7   6   5   4   3   2

We acknowledge the patience and endurance of our families as we locked ourselves away from all but the pursuit of research to accomplish this goal.

To Irene and Everett N. Strawn, Jr.

R.M.M.S.

To Wayne, Bonnie Sue, Deborah, Ginger, "Rocky," Matthew, Denis, Angel, Benjamin, Katie, Joani, Chelsea, Sarah, Carrie, Nina, Kristin, Kelli and Kori.

B.P.F.S.

CONTENTS

PREFACE

Change in critical care is essential. It is required, and we who practice in the critical care setting must be open to those changes—in technology, in methodology, in knowledge base, and in the way we deliver care.

Although the primary focus of *Ready Reference for Critical Care, Second Edition,* remains the same, we have included updated information on ventilators, pacemakers, and new ACLS algorithms in this edition. Newer medications have been included and a new medication format is introduced. This book should prove more worthwhile than ever in orienting, training, and monitoring the activity of unlicensed assistive personnel.

This book is not an original work. It is, instead, a compilation of all the scraps and tidbits of information that have been tacked or taped to medication room walls or "stashed" in forgotten nooks and crannies. We have attempted to put it all together, concisely, in a single volume.

We have researched, as carefully as possible, literature obtained from manufacturers, researchers, developers, and educators. Every attempt has been made to comply with recommendations for dosages, usage, and availability.

It should, however, be understood that some *differences,* regional or institutional, will be noted. It must also be recognized that all information in this work is to be applied, *solely,* to adult patients. *No* information is included that concerns either pediatric or pregnant patients. As is also to be expected, changes occur in clinical practice and research almost daily. Whenever using drugs, equipment, or procedures, it is imperative that you be completely familiar with accepted standards of manufacturers and producers. Always check package inserts and manufacturers' references.

A work of this magnitude could never be accomplished without much assistance. Many people gave time, energy, and expertise in the preparation of the first edition, and we wish to recognize their contributions.

Dr. William H. Hill, MD, PhD, offered technical assistance as well as emotional support. Libby Whitley, RN, MSN, CCRN, spent many hours answering questions related to coronary care. Rose Weatherly, RN, CNN, and Martha Perrett, RN, provided us with materials and information on kidney disease and dialysis. Joseph Spence, BS, RPh, provided answers for numerous questions related to pharmaceutical agents. Velda Graphenreed, RN, spent many hours collecting original monitor strips.

Dick Reid of Medtronic Pacing Systems assisted us in the research on the pacemaker section. Dennis Battersby of Amicon Division of W.R. Grace Company provided information on ECMO and dialytic therapy. Judy Atkins of Kabivitrum Incorporated provided us with information on amino acids and fat emulsions.

In addition, we express sincerest gratitude to those persons who have contributed to the genesis and upgrade of this book. We have attempted to take sound principles and to translate them into clear, practical, "do-able" strategies.

Of course, we are obliged to many others who have answered questions, or in some instances, asked questions that have spurred us on to further research on a particular subject. We also thank those persons.

It is our hope that the revisions in *Ready Reference for Critical Care, Second Edition,* will be of value to *all* critical care providers, and that you, as the reader, will find it useful to your practice.

CARDIAC EVALUATION
AND MANAGEMENT

HEART SOUNDS

Sound	Origin	Auscultatory Site	Ear Piece/ Pt. Position	Pitch	Timing	Respiratory Variation
S$_1$	*Normal sound* Closing of mitral and tricuspid valves Corresponds to ventricular depolarization	Apex LLSB (mitral area)	Diaphragm Patient supine	High	Beginning of systole	None
Split S$_1$	Right bundle branch block (RBBB) Mitral stenosis	Apex LLSB	Diaphragm Patient supine	High	Beginning of systole	None
S$_2$	*Normal sound* Closing of aortic and pulmonic valves Corresponds to ventricular repolarization	2nd ICS, RSB Aortic area; louder than S$_1$ at this site	Diaphragm Patient supine	High	End of systole	None
Split S$_2$ (physiologic)	*Normal* in children and young adults	2nd ICS, LSB	Diaphragm Patient supine	High	End of systole	↑ inspiration Absent on expiration
Wide S$_2$ (persistent)	Late closure of pulmonic valve Early closure of aortic valve Atrial septal defect	2nd ICS, LSB	Diaphragm Patient supine	High	End of systole	↑ inspiration ↓ expiration

	Left ventricular failure RBBB Pulmonic stenosis Hypertension					
Reversed S$_2$ (paradoxical)	Delayed left ventricular systole Aortic valve closes after the pulmonic valve	2nd ICS, LSB	Diaphragm Patient supine	High	End of systole	Heard on expiration
Reversed S$_2$	Left ventricular failure Left bundle branch block (LBBB) Myocardial infarction Aortic stenosis Hypertension					
Split S$_2$ (fixed)	Split of pulmonic-aortic elements Pulmonic stenosis Atrial septal defect	2nd ICS, LSB	Diaphragm Patient supine	High	End of systole	None
S$_3$ (right ventricular origin)	Abnormal ventricular filling pressure Emphysema	LLSB or xyphoid	Bell Patient supine left lateral position (fainter when sitting or standing)	Low Dull	Early diastole (follows second sound)	↑ inspiration

Sound	Origin	Auscultatory Site	Ear Piece/ Pt. Position	Pitch	Timing	Respiratory Variation
S$_3$ (left ventricular origin) Ventricular gallop Physiological 3rd heart sound	Abnormal ventricular filling pressure Congestive heart failure (CHF) Third trimester pregnancy Common in children or adults over 50	Apex	Bell Patient supine or left lateral position	Low Dull	Early diastole (after S$_2$)	↑ expiration
S$_4$ (right ventricular origin) Atrial diastolic gallop	Atrial filling against resistance from decreased *right* ventricular compliance Myocardial disease Coronary artery disease (CAD) Pulmonic stenosis	LLSB	Bell Patient supine or left lateral position	Low Dull	Late in diastole Before S$_1$	↑ inspiration
S$_4$ (left ventricular origin) Atrial diastolic gallop	Atrial filling against resistance from decreased *left* ventricular compliance CAD	Apex	Bell Patient supine or left lateral position	Low	Late in diastole just prior to S$_1$	↑ expiration ↓ inspiration

	Primary myocardial disease Aortic stenosis Hypertension Corresponds to atrial depolarization **Fourth heart sound often is loudest during initial stage of MI or during episodes of acute pain. Sound becomes fainter as patient improves.**					
Ejection click	Opening of the semilunar valves (aortic or pulmonic) Valvular disease Rapid ejection through a normal valve **Distinguish from S_4, which has a low pitch, "thudding" quality, and is heard in a limited area (usually the apex).**	Heard in many areas including the apex	Diaphragm Patient supine	High/sharp	Onset of ventricular ejection, just after S_1	None

Sound	Origin	Auscultatory Site	Ear Piece/ Pt. Position	Pitch	Timing	Respiratory Variation
Systolic nonejection click	Prolapse or backward motion of mitral valve leaflet during systole **To differentiate from second heart sound, listen over the Base and identify S_1 and S_2. Then gradually move the stethoscope down the sternal border until the click accompanies each beat.**	LLSB (sometimes confused with S_2)	Diaphragm Patient supine	High (snapping sound)	Mid to late systolic Precedes S_2	None

Note: LLSB = left lateral sternal border; ICS = intercostal space; RSB = right sternal border; LSB = left sternal border.

CLASSIFICATION OF MURMURS

CLASS†

I	Very faint; easily missed
II	Barely audible
III	Easily heard
IV	Loud; may be associated with a thrill
V	Louder with an obvious thrill
VI	Very loud with a thrill; may be heard with the stethoscope just off the chest wall

---

†Six-point grading scale; sounds classified as IV, V, or VI can be felt or palpated.

Condition	Timing	Duration	Pitch	Quality	Auscultatory Site	Radiation	Noted Changes	EKG Variance
Mitral insufficiency	Systolic	Pansystolic/ejection	High	Blowing/plateau	Apex; 5th–6th ICS left MCL	Left axilla	↑ with squatting	Abnormal P wave; left atrial enlargement
Mitral stenosis	Diastolic	Mid-diastolic/presystolic	Low	Rumbling/crescendo	Apex; 5th ICS LMCL	Toward axilla	↑ in left lateral position or exercise	Atrial fibrillation
Tricuspid insufficiency	Systolic	Midsystolic	Medium/high	Blowing/plateau	4th LICS	RSB, toward the apex	↑ with respiration	Peaked P wave; right heart enlargement indicating axis deviation
Tricuspid stenosis	Diastolic	Early diastolic	Low	Rumbling/crescendo–decrescendo	4th LICS	Apex, xyphoid	↑ with inspiration	Peak P wave; right atrial enlargement
Aortic insufficiency	Diastolic	Early diastolic	High	Blowing/decrescendo	4th LICS 3rd LICS 2nd RICS	Apex, LSB	↑ with leaning forward and with expiration	Increased QRS and ST-T depression; left ventricular enlargement

Aortic stenosis	Systolic	Midsystolic	Medium/high	Harsh/crescendo–decrescendo	2nd RICS	Neck, upper back, right carotid, apex	↑ with sitting, supine position, squatting, or holding breath	Large S waves in right precordial leads Large R waves in left precordial leads ST depression, inverted T waves
Pulmonic insufficiency	Diastolic	Early diastolic	High	Blowing/decrescendo	2nd LICS	Toward the sternum/apex	↑ with inspiration	May be normal Right axis deviation indicating ventricular enlargement
Pulmonic stenosis	Systolic	Systolic ejection	Medium/high	Harsh/crescendo	2nd LICS	Left shoulder, left side of neck, back	↑ with inspiration	May be normal Right axis deviation indicating ventricular enlargement

Condition	Timing	Duration	Pitch	Quality	Auscultatory Site	Radiation	Noted Changes	EKG Variance
Ventricular septal defects	Systolic	Pansystolic/ ejection	High	Blowing/ plateau	4th LICS	Toward RSB	None	Left ventricular hypertrophy
Atrial septal defects	Systolic/ diastolic	Continuous	Medium/ low	Crescendo/ decrescendo	2nd LICS/ 4th LICS	LLSB Murmur may vary, depending on the direction of the shunt (R → L or L → R)	↑ inspiration	May be normal Atrial fibrillation Varying degrees of RBBB Right ventricular hypertrophy
Idiopathic hypertrophic sub-aortic stenosis	Systolic	Ejection	High	Crescendo/ decrescendo	2nd RICS 3rd RICS 4th RICS	Neck, upper back, apex	↑ with inspiration, Valsalva maneuver	Left ventricular hypertrophy ST-T wave abnormality Left anterior hemiblock Ventricular arrhythmias Atrial fibrillation

Coarctation of the aorta	Systolic	Ejection	Medium	Crescendo	Left mid-back be-tween scapulae	Neck	None	Left ventri-ular hyper-trophy
Patent duc-tus arterio-sus (aortic-atrial shunt)	Systolic/ diastolic	Continuous	High	May vary	2nd LICS	Neck	None	Left ventric-ular hyper-trophy if shunt is large

Note: MCL = midclavical line; LMCL = left midclavical line; ICS = intercostal space; RICS = right intercostal space; LICS = left intercostal space; RSB = right sternal border; LSB = left sternal border.

CONTINUOUS BEDSIDE MONITORING

LEAD PLACEMENT

	Lead Placement	Essentials of Lead Placement
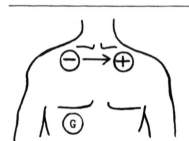 **Figure 1.1** Lead I	**Lead I** • Positive electrode below left clavicle • Negative electrode below right clavicle	• Less artifact noted in mechanically ventilated patients • P and QRS usually positive
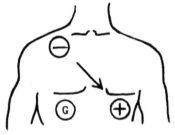 **Figure 1.2** Lead II	**Lead II** • Positive electrode below left pectoral muscle • Negative electrode below right clavicle	• Most popular monitoring lead • Good P and R waveforms • Facilitates detection of QRS axis shift • Poor differentiation of the origin of BBB • Unable to distinguish ventricular ectopy from aberration

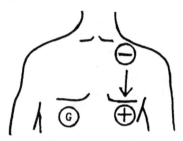

Figure 1.3   Lead III

Lead III
- Positive electrode below left pectoral muscle
- Negative electrode below left clavicle

- Identifies the polarity of the retrograde P′
- QRS may be diphasic

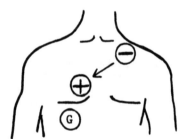

Figure 1.4   MCL₁ (Modified V₁)

MCL$_1$ (Modified V$_1$)
- Positive electrode to right of sternum in 4th ICS
- Negative electrode near left shoulder (outer third of left clavicle)

- Facilitates countershock
- Contrast left ventricular ectopy (QRS negative) and right ventricular ectopy (QRS positive)
- Allows differentiation between VT and aberration
- Best lead for distinguishing BBB
- Detects improper placement of pacing catheter
- Distinct P waves in right-chest leads
- Fails to perceive shifts of axis

Lead Placement	Essentials of Lead Placement

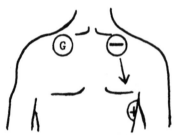

MCL$_6$ (Modified V$_6$)

* Positive electrode
  left midaxillary line in 5th ICS
* Negative electrode
  near left shoulder (outer third of
  left clavicle)

* Identifies supraventricular
  tachycardia
* Differentiates BBB
* Highlights right ventricular
  pacemaker complexes
* Impedes countershock

Figure 1.5 MCL$_6$ (Modified V$_6$)

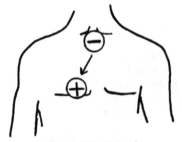

S$_5$ Lead

* Positive electrode
  5th RICS close to sternum
* Negative electrode
  on manubrium

* Greatly magnifies P waves
* Facilitates diagnosis of atrial
  tachycardia with 2:1 block
* Takes place of esophageal or atrial
  leads

Figure 1.6 S$_5$ Lead

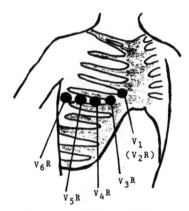

Right Precordial Leads

- Placed in same anatomic configuration as opposite left chest leads
- Lead V_4R in 5th ICS, midclavicular line
- Lead V_3R equidistant between V_1 (V_2R and V_4R)
- Lead V_5R in same horizontal plane as V_4 in anterior axillary line
- Lead V_6R in same horizontal line as V_4 and V_5 at midaxillary line
- To gain electrocardiographic information about right ventricular disorders, atrial arrhythmias, and congenital heart disease.

Figure 1.7   Right Precordial Leads

Note: Ground electrode is usually positioned anywhere, but most commonly below the right pectoral muscle.
BBB = bundle branch block; ICS = intercostal space; RICS = right intercostal space.

CARDIAC RHYTHMS

Normal Sinus Rhythm (NSR)

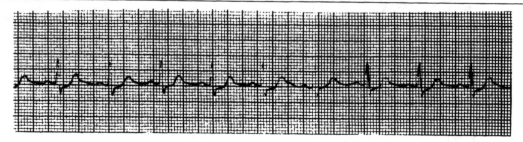

Figure 1.8 Normal Sinus Rhythm

Characteristics
- Rate: 60–100 beats per minute (BPM)
- Rhythm: regular
- P waves: present; normal (smoothly rounded; upright in leads I, II, and aVF; inverted in aVR)
- PR interval: 0.12–0.20 sec
- QRS: normally less than 0.12 sec
- Conduction: each P wave followed by one QRS

Sinus Arrhythmia

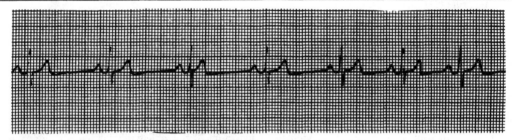

Figure 1.9 Sinus Arrhythmia

Etiology
- Vagal inhibition causing irregularity of sinus pacemaker
- Digitalis toxicity, increased intracranial pressure (ICP), inferior wall myocardial infarction (MI)
- Variation of NSR related to respiratory cycle

Characteristics
- Rate: variable
- Rhythm: slightly irregular
- P waves: normal; PR interval varies
- QRS: usually normal

Nursing/Medical Intervention
- None

Atropine may abolish the irregular rhythm or increase the rate.

Sinus Tachycardia (ST)

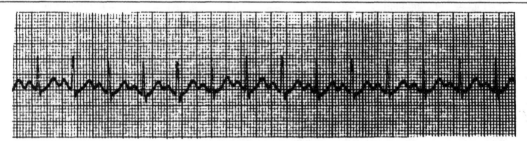

Figure 1.10   Sinus Tachycardia

Etiology

- Exercise, anxiety, fever, pain, dehydration, anemia, hyperthyroidism, hypovolemia, caffeine
- MI
- Pulmonary embolus (PE)
- Mitral stenosis
- Vagolytic/sympathetic drugs

Characteristics

- Rate: 100–150 BPM
- Rhythm: regular
- Every QRS preceded by a P

Nursing/Medical Intervention

- Document dysrhythmia
- Monitor hemodynamic parameters
- Treat underlying cause

Wandering Atrial Pacemaker

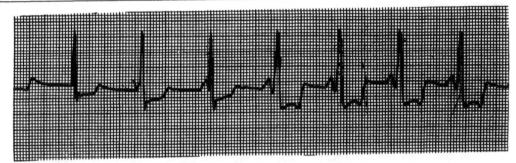

Figure 1.11 Wandering Atrial Pacemaker

Etiology
- Inflammation of SA node (rheumatic fever)
- Digitalis toxicity
- Sick sinus syndrome (SSS)

Characteristics
- Rate: variable; <100 BPM
- Rhythm: slightly irregular with changing morphology; **never** premature; PR interval varies
- QRS: normal

Nursing/Medical Intervention
- Detect and document dysrhythmia; differentiate from premature atrial contractions
- Monitor pulse, blood pressure, and peripheral pulses
- Monitor cardiac output and sensorium
- Treat bradycardia if present and patient is symptomatic

Use Digitalis with caution.

Sinus Bradycardia

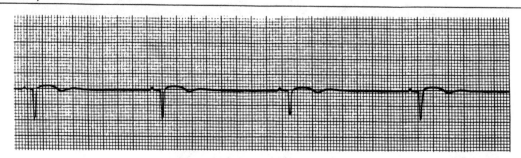

Figure 1.12   Sinus Bradycardia

Etiology
- Normal variant in athletes, some healthy adults
- Increased vagal tone (vomiting, straining)
- Increased ICP
- Digitalis/Quinidine toxicity
- Sympatholytic drugs/beta-blockers
- Hyperkalemia
- MI

Characteristics
- Rate: <60 BPM
- Rhythm: regular
- P waves: normal; PR interval normal or prolonged
- QRS: normal

Nursing/Medical Intervention
- Document dysrhythmia
- Maintain patient airway
- Monitor hemodynamic parameters for reduction in cardiac output, hypotension, weak peripheral pulses, progressive CHF
- Evaluate neurological status
- If asymptomatic: no treatment
- If symptomatic:
  –*atropine*—0.5 mg every 5 min for a total of 2.0 mg
  –*isuprel*—2–10 mcg/min
  –*pacemaker*—if indicated

Refer to ACLS algorithm (Fig. 1.43).

Sinus Block

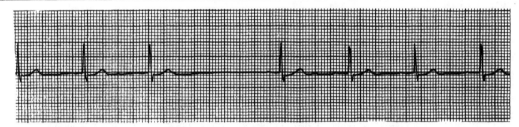

Figure 1.13   Sinus Block

Etiology

- Increased vagal tone
- Ischemia
- Coronary artery disease (CAD)
- Infectious myocarditis
- Digitalis/Quinidine toxicity

Characteristics

- Rate: flat line (exactly the length of one or more R–R intervals)
- Rhythm: normal rhythm will resume at a predictable spot
- P waves: none
- QRS: absent
- SA node fails to activate the atria

Nursing/Medical Intervention

- If asymptomatic, no treatment necessary
- Treat bradycardia
- Treat underlying cause

Administer atropine to increase the rate.

Sinus Pause

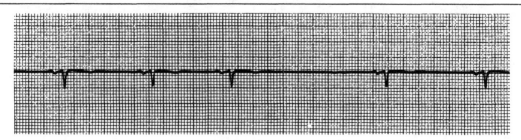

Figure 1.14   Sinus Pause

Etiology
- Vagal stimulation
- Digitalis/Quinidine toxicity
- Degenerative heart disease
- Anoxic sinus node

Characteristics
- Rate: flat line *less* than 3 sec
- Rhythm: R–R cycle interrupted
- P waves: none
- QRS: absent
- Failure of SA node to initiate an impulse

Nursing/Medical Intervention
- If asymptomatic, no treatment necessary
- Treat bradycardia
- Treat underlying cause

Sinus Arrest

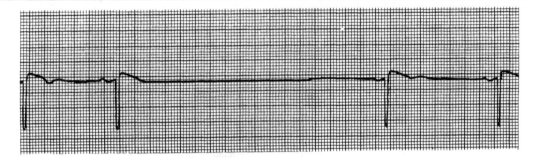

Figure 1.15 Sinus Arrest

Etiology
- Vagal stimulation
- Digitalis/Quinidine toxicity
- Degenerative heart disease
- Anoxic sinus node

Characteristics
- Rate: flat line *greater* than 3 sec
- Rhythm: R–R cycle interrupted
- P waves: none
- QRS: absent
- Failure of SA node to initiate an impulse

Nursing/Medical Intervention
- Treat underlying cause
- Pacemaker for recurrent episodes

If hemodynamic compromise is evident, atropine may be indicated.

Atrial Escape Beats[†]

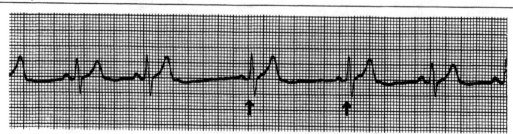

Figure 1.16   Atrial Escape Beats

Etiology
- Increased vagal tone
- Hypoxia
- Ischemia
- Degenerative heart disease
- MI
- Digitalis/quinidine toxicity

Characteristics
- Rate: variable; usually slow
- Rhythm: irregular
- P waves: precede every QRS; morphology may vary; normal PR interval
- QRS: normal
- Impulse arises in atria, not SA node

Nursing/Medical Intervention
- Detect and document dysrhythmia
- Administer O_2
- Treat symptoms (syncope, lightheadedness)
- If patient symptomatic, IV atropine may be indicated
- If atropine ineffective, use Isuprel infusion
- Place in supine position and consider external pacing
- Treat underlying cause

[†]If condition persists for more than 3 beats, it is called *atrial escape rhythm.*

Junctional Escape Beats[†]

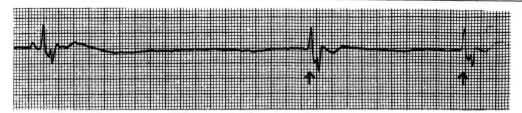

Figure 1.17 Junctional Escape Beats

Etiology
- Hypoxia
- Ischemia
- CAD
- Infectious myocarditis
- MI (inferior wall)
- Digitalis/Quinidine toxicity

Characteristics
- Rate: 40–60 BPM
- Rhythm: regular; produced by a single ectopic pacemaker
- P waves: absent or variable; PR interval altered
- QRS: normal
- Junctional escape beats occur by default
- Pacemaker above the AV node fails to fire or AV node blocks impulse

Nursing/Medical Intervention
- Detect and document rhythm by default
- Evaluate blood pressure, skin color/temperature, and level of consciousness
- Attempt to determine cause of dysrhythmia
- Treat presenting symptoms
- Treat underlying cause

[†]If condition persists for more than 3 beats, it is called *junctional escape rhythm* or *idiojunctional rhythm.*

Ventricular Escape Beats[†]

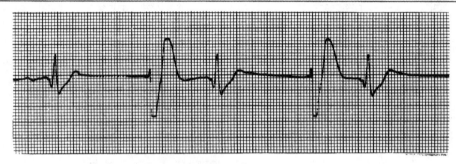

Figure 1.18   Ventricular Escape Beats

Etiology

- Hypoxia
- Myocardial ischemia
- Shock
- Digitalis/quinidine toxicity
- Electrolyte derangements (monitor serum potassium)

Characteristics

- Rate: <40 BPM
- Rhythm: regular if produced by a single pacemaker
- P waves: usually absent; if present, dissociated from QRS (AV dissociation)
- QRS: wide and bizarre; may be opposite from expected deflection
- T wave may be oppositely deflected

Nursing/Medical Intervention

- Detect and document dysrhythmia
- Evaluate level of consciousness/sensorium
- Monitor hemodynamic parameters
- If pulseless and apneic, start CPR
- Oxygen
- Pacemaker
- Monitor for emerging secondary dysrhythmias

Ventricular escape complexes or rhythms should not be suppressed.

[†]Also referred to as *idioventricular rhythm*.

First Degree (Incomplete) AV Block

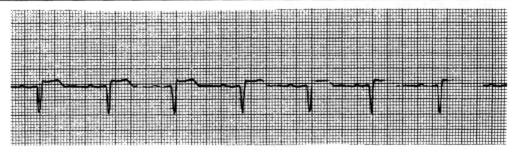

Figure 1.19   First Degree AV Block

Etiology
- Increased vagal tone
- Inferior wall MI
- Subacute bacterial endocarditis
- Myocarditis
- Chronic heart disease
- Drugs that slow AV node conduction (digitalis, beta-blockers, calcium channel blockers)

Characteristics
- Rate: 60–100 BPM
- Rhythm: regular
- P waves: Normal; PR interval >0.20 sec
- QRS: normal
- Partial block at the AV node
- May be a normal variant

Nursing/Medical Intervention
- If dysrhythmia produces a slow rate and is symptomatic, follow same plan as for sinus bradycardia
- Treat underlying cause
- Observe for increase in AV block (may result in loss of "atrial kick," decreased ventricular ejection, and cardiac output)

Administer Digitalis cautiously.

Second Degree (Mobitz Type I—Wenckebach) AV Block

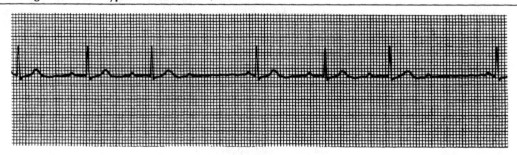

Figure 1.20 Second degree AV Block (Type I)

Etiology
- Vagal stimulation
- Inferior wall MI
- Rheumatic fever
- Digitalis toxicity
- Beta-blockers
- Verapamil ingestion

Characteristics
- Rate: within normal range
- Rhythm: atrial—regular; ventricular—irregular with "cluster" of repetitive patterns
- P waves: normal; PR lengthens with each successive beat until a beat is dropped
- QRS: normal

Nursing/Medical Intervention
- Detect and document dysrhythmia
- Treat underlying cause
- Observe for higher degree of AV block
- Atropine or Isuprel if patient is symptomatic
- Discontinue Digitalis

Second Degree (Mobitz Type II—Fixed or Varied Ratio) AV Block

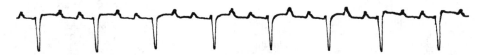

Figure 1.21   Second Degree AV Block (Type II)

Etiology
- Anteroseptal MI
- CAD
- Degenerative disease of conduction system (His-Purkinje)
- AV node ischemia
- Digitalis toxicity

Characteristics
- Rate: atrial—within normal range; ventricular—may be slow
- Rhythm: irregular with varying degrees of block
- P waves: P–P interval constant with dropped QRS complexes
- QRS: intermittently absent; may be abnormally wide

Nursing/Medical Intervention
- Detect and document dysrhythmia
- Atropine if patient hemodynamically unstable
- Isuprel[†]
- Pacemaker
- Discontinue Digitalis

[†]Consider the oxygen supply–demand relationship.

Third Degree (Complete) AV Block

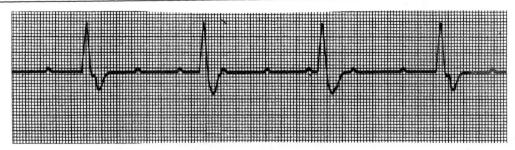

Figure 1.22   Third Degree AV Block

Etiology
- Acute MI
- Digitalis toxicity
- Ischemic heart disease
- Degenerative disease of conduction system
- Infectious disease of myocardium

Characteristics
- Rate: atrial rate—greater than ventricular; ventricular rate—usually <40
- Rhythm: atrial—regular; ventricular—regular; rhythms are independent, i.e., have no association
- P waves: normal with varying PR intervals
- QRS: variable; narrow if pacemaker junctional; wide if pacemaker ventricular

Nursing/Medical Intervention
- Identify absence of AV conduction
- Evaluate signs/symptoms of slow heart rate: confusion, light-headedness, fatigue, and CHF
- Monitor hemodynamic parameters
- Ascertain possibility of drug toxicity
- Monitor tolerance to dysrhythmia
- Atropine[†]
- Isuprel
- Transvenous pacemaker

[†]Atropine is not usually effective in restoring AV conduction but may produce therapeutic effect.

AV Dissociation[†]

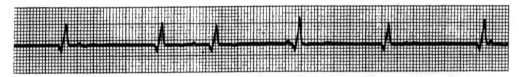

Figure 1.23A   AV Dissociation Resulting from Slowing of the Sinus Rate
Reprinted with permission from Marriott, HJL: Practical Electrocardiography, 8th ed. Baltimore: Williams & Wilkins, 1988.

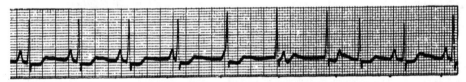

Figure 1.23B   AV Dissociation Resulting from Increased Automaticity of a Subsidiary Pacemaker
Reprinted with permission from Marriott, HJL: Practical Electrocardiography, 8th ed. Baltimore: Williams & Wilkins, 1988.

AV Dissociation[†] (*continued*)

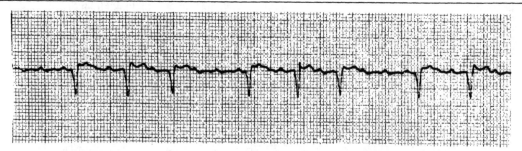

Figure 1.23C   AV Dissociation Resulting from AV Block

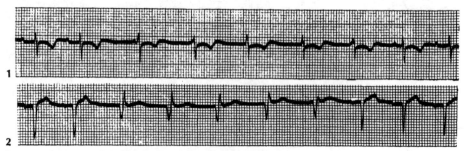

Figure 1.23D   AV Dissociation Resulting from Combination/Deviation of the Previous Disorders: **(1)** Sinus Arrhythmia with a Rate of About 58 Beats/Min; **(2)** Nonconducted PAC with a Long Enough Cycle for an Accelerated Idioventricular Rhythm to Intercede

Reprinted with permission from Marriott, HJL: Practical Electrocardiography, 8th ed. Baltimore: Williams & Wilkins, 1988.

Etiology

- Athletic heart
- Digitalis intoxication
- Acute MI
- Postcardiac surgery
- Rheumatic heart disease
- Degenerative cardiac disease
- Can result from one or four basic disorders:
  - *Slowing of sinus rate* to <40–60; inherent junctional rate (AV dissociation by default)
  - *Increased automaticity of a subsidiary pacemaker*—junctional/ventricular tachycardia; accelerated idiojunctional/idioventricular rhythm
  - *Atrioventricular block*—atria and ventricles beat independently; AV block just *one* cause of AV dissociation; AV dissociation not always complete AV block
  - *Combination of deviations,* from the previous disorders

Characteristics

- Rate: varies according to etiology
- Rhythm: may be regular or irregular; atrial rhythm independent of ventricular rhythm
- P waves: configuration varies; dissociated from QRS; PR interval not measured in AV dissociation
- QRS: configuration varies depending on origin of impulse

Nursing/Medical Intervention

- Identify and document dysrhythmia
- Monitor hemodynamic parameters
- Assess and evaluate orientation, skin color/temperature, and peripheral pulses
- Identify irregular cannon waves
- Note any changes in S_1 heart sounds
- Treat underlying cause
- Treat observable symptoms

---

†Not recognized as a dysrhythmia. Not a primary disturbance, it occurs as a secondary phenomenon in response to a basic disorder.

Right Bundle Branch Block (RBBB)

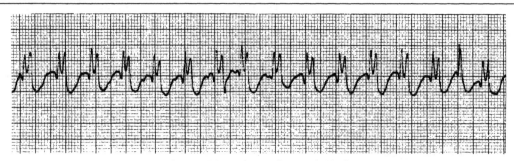

Figure 1.24   Right Bundle Branch Block

Etiology
- Degenerative or sclerotic aortic or tricuspid valves
- Anteroseptal MI
- Diseases of right ventricle
- Swan–Ganz catheter insertion
- CAD

Characteristics
- Prolongation of QRS complex: $\geq$0.12 sec
- Triphasic QRS complex
  V_1 rSR′
  V_6 qRs′
- Wide terminal R′ in V_1
- Wide terminal s in V_6

Incomplete **RBBB exhibits a QRS <0.12 sec.**

Nursing/Medical Intervention
- Monitor RBBB in V_1 or MCL_1
- Monitor hemodynamic parameters; clinical symptoms not usually noted
- No treatment indicated
- Electrical pacing not usually indicated

Left Bundle Branch Block (LBBB)

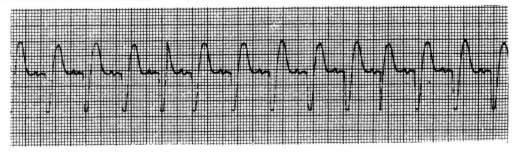

Figure 1.25   Left Bundle Branch Block

Etiology

- Ischemia
- Mechanical compression of its origin
- Organic heart disease
- CAD
- Anteroseptal/anterolateral MI

Characteristics

- Prolongation of QRS complex: ≥0.12 sec
- Wide R in V_6—may be "slurred" or notched
- QS or rS in V_1

Incomplete **LBBB exhibits a normal QRS duration.**

Nursing/Medical Intervention

- Monitor MCL_1, MCL_6, V_1, and V_6 to determine presence of LBBB
- With acute anteroseptal or anterolateral MI, LBBB may develop
- Monitor for worsening of heart block in the presence of ventricular myocardial injury
- No pharmacological intervention necessary
- Electrical pacing in selected situations

Premature Atrial Contractions (PACs)—Atrial Extrasystole

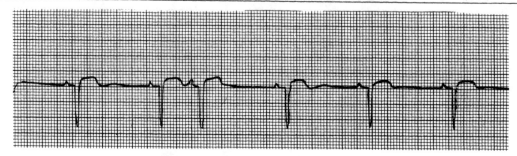

Figure 1.26   Premature Atrial Contractions

Etiology

- Acute MI
- Congestive heart failure (CHF)
- Ischemic heart disease
- CAD
- PE
- Electrolyte imbalance
- Digitalis toxicity
- Anxiety
- Aminophyllin/adrenergic drugs
- Caffeine
- May be a normal variant

Characteristics

- Rate: may be within normal range
- Rhythm: irregular because of premature P wave and resulting QRS
- P waves: different from the sinus P; PR interval ≥0.12 sec
- QRS: normal if present; may be blocked
- Noncompensatory pause may be noted

Nursing/Medical Intervention

- Detect and document irregular pulse
- Validate irregularity by ECG
- Assess for symptoms such as hypotension, light-headedness, or palpitations
- Assess for CHF symptoms and evaluate respiratory status
- No treatment if asymptomatic
- Treat underlying cause
- If increasing in frequency (5–6 BPM), Digitalis, quinidine, or propranolol may be indicated

Atrial Fibrillation (AF)

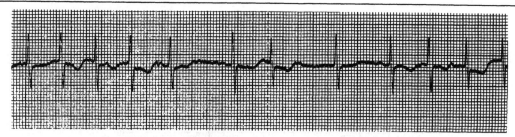

Figure 1.27 Atrial Fibrillation

Etiology
- Hypertensive cardiovascular disease
- Mitral valve disease
- Ischemic heart disease
- Hyperthyroidism
- CHF
- Postcoronary bypass or valve replacement surgery

Characteristics
- Rate: atrial—too rapid to determine; ventricular—variable, count for 1 min
- Rhythm: irregular—both atrial and ventricular
- P waves: chaotic; not identifiable; PR interval not measurable
- QRS: usually normal

Nursing/Medical Intervention
- Detect and document dysrhythmia
- Monitor for diminished cardiac output
- Monitor pulse and blood pressure
- Evaluate quality of peripheral pulses
- Monitor sensorium
- Assess for CHF signs/symptoms
- Cardioversion if AF is new onset (<1 yr)
- Digitalis
- Quinidine (after digitalization)
- Beta-blockers
- Procainamide
- Diuretics (for CHF)
- Anticoagulants (prophylactically)

Atrial Flutter (AF)

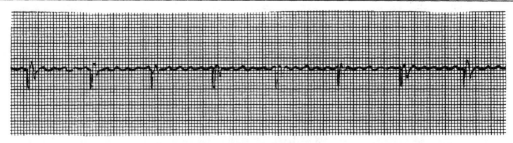

Figure 1.28 Atrial Flutter

Etiology
- CAD
- Rheumatic heart disease
- PE
- Acute MI
- Pericarditis/myocarditis
- Cardiomyopathy
- Wolff–Parkinson–White (WPW) syndrome
- Postcoronary revascularization

Characteristics
- Rate: atrial—250–350 BPM; ventricular—depends on degree of AV block
- Rhythm: atrial—regular; ventricular—regular or irregular
- P waves: "saw tooth"; appear in multiples before each QRS; PR interval not measurable
- QRS: usually normal

Nursing/Medical Intervention
- Detect and document dysrhythmia
- Monitor for signs of decreased cardiac output
- Monitor pulse and blood pressure
- Monitor sensorium
- Assess for CHF signs/symptoms
- Verapamil
- Esmolol
- Digitalization
- Quinidine
- Synchronized cardioversion
- Atrial overdrive pacing

Atrial Tachycardia (Nonparoxysmal, with Block)[†]

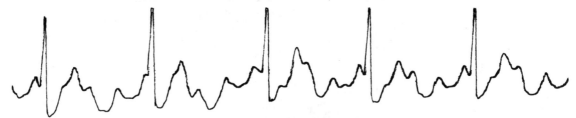

Figure 1.29   Atrial Tachycardia (with Block)

Etiology
- Increased atrial automaticity
- MI
- Digitalis toxicity
- Hypokalemia
- COPD
- Hypoxia
- Amphetamines
- Alcohol ingestion

Characteristics
- Rate: atrial—100–200 BPM; ventricular—less than atrial
- Rhythm: atrial—regular; ventricular—regular or irregular
- P waves: small (visible), uniform/multiform; PR interval normal or prolonged
- QRS: usually normal (not every P wave produces a QRS)

Nursing/Medical Intervention
- Detect and document dysrhythmia
- Monitor pulse and blood pressure
- Monitor potassium and digoxin levels
- Beta-blockers
- Calcium channel blockers
- Digitalis (if serum level within normal range)
- Valsalva maneuver

[†]Occurrence of three or more consecutive PACs is considered atrial tachycardia, which may be confused with ST (rate: 150–160 BPM). In ST, P waves are uniform, regular, and slightly larger.

Paroxysmal Supraventricular Tachycardia (PSVT)—Reentrant/Reciprocating Impulse

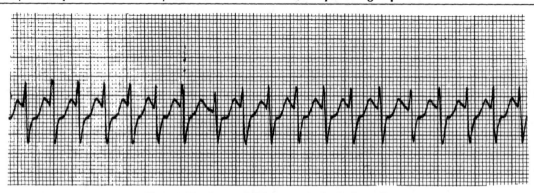

Figure 1.30   Paroxysmal Supraventricular Tachycardia

Etiology

- AV nodal reentry
- Sympathomimetic drugs
- Mitral valve prolapse
- Fever, sepsis, hyperthyroidism
- Myocarditis
- Cardiomyopathy
- Caffeine, alcohol, tobacco

Characteristics

- Rate: 150–250 BPM
- Rhythm: regular
- P waves: may be unidentifiable; if visible, have relationship with QRS; PR interval not usually measurable
- QRS: normal

PSVT: Onset and termination are abrupt.

Nursing/Medical Intervention

- Detect and document a rapid, regular pulse
- Assess for signs/symptoms of diminished cardiac output; hypotension, light-headedness, diaphoresis, confusion, or diminished level of consciousness
- Evaluate for CHF signs/symptoms
- Reflex vagal stimulation
  – carotid sinus massage
  – valsalva maneuver
- Verapamil
- Adenocard
- Digitalis
- Beta-blockers
- Type I antiarrhythmics
- Synchronized cardioversion

Refer to ACLS algorithm (Fig. 1.44).

Premature Junctional Contractions (PJCs)—Junctional Extrasystole

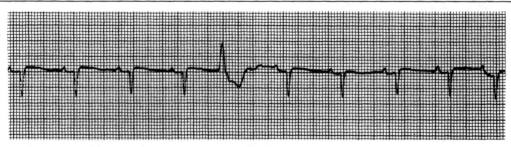

Figure 1.31   Premature Junctional Contractions

Etiology
- Increased automaticity
- Ischemia
- Digitalis toxicity
- CHF
- MI
- Rheumatic heart disease
- Caffeine
- Amphetamines

Characteristics
- Rate: variable; normal range
- Rhythm: irregular
- P wave: may be before, within, *or* after the QRS; PR interval ≤0.10 sec; if after the QRS, R–P′ ≤0.20 sec

P′ preceding the QRS *is early*. If P′ is not early, consider PVC (pages 45–47).

Nursing/Medical Intervention
- Detect and document dysrhythmia; document frequency of the PJCs
- Evaluate signs/symptoms of diminished cardiac output
- Treat underlying cause
- Quinidine
- Disopyramide
- May need to discontinue Digitalis if patient is taking it

Junctional Tachycardia (JT)[†]

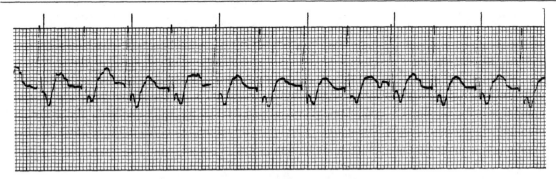

Figure 1.32 Junctional Tachycardia

[†]Occurrence of three or more consecutive PJCs is considered junctional tachycardia; it is rarely encountered.

Etiology

- Enhanced automaticity
- Myocardial ischemia
- MI
- Myocarditis
- Cardiomyopathy
- Digitalis toxicity

Characteristics

- Rate: 100–200 BPM; gradually accelerates
- Rhythm: regular; ratio 1:1
- P waves: buried in the QRS or in T waves of preceding beat
- QRS: usually normal

Nursing/Medical Intervention

- Detect and document dysrhythmia
- Evaluate patient response to reduced ventricular filling time and loss of atrial kick
- Monitor blood pressure, skin color/temperature, and level of consciousness
- Monitor for CHF signs/symptoms
- Treat underlying cause
- Carotid sinus massage
- Valsalva maneuver
- Digitalis
- Propranolol
- Esmolol

Premature Ventricular Contractions (PVCs)

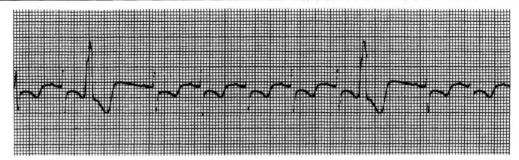

Figure 1.33A Unifocal PVCs

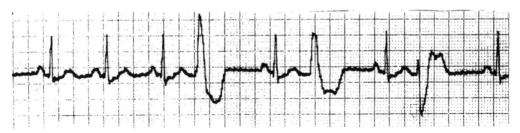

Figure 1.33B Multifocal PVCs

Premature Ventricular Contractions (*continued*)

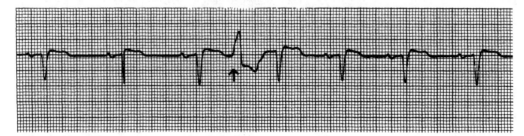

Figure 1.33C   Interpolated PVC

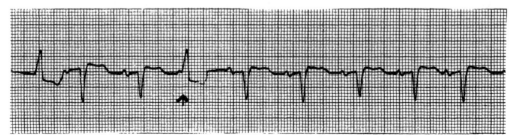

Figure 1.33D   End-Diastolic PVC

Etiology

- CAD
- Enhanced automaticity
- Reentry mechanism
- Digitalis, amphetamines, theophyllin, adrenergics, Isuprel, dopamine
- Tobacco, caffeine, alcohol
- Hypoxia, acidosis
- Electrolyte imbalance
- Increased preload/afterload
- Acute asthma
- Emotional stress
- Exercise

Characteristics

- Rate: may be any rate
- Rhythm: usually irregular
- P waves: PVCs not preceded by P' wave; PR interval not present
- QRS: premature; ≥0.12 sec; wide and aberrant
- Usually has compensatory pause
- Complex must be early
- Interpolated PVC "sandwiched" between two sinus beats; R–R interval constant; PR of succeeding complex may be longer (see Fig. 1.33C)
- End-diastolic PVC preceded by a P wave (P not early; if P early, consider PJC); ectopic beat late enough to occur *after* sinus P wave
- May occur singly, in pairs (bigeminy), triples (trigeminy), or any combination of numbers
- Potentially lethal in couplets, runs, and salvos; multifocal and R on T
- Fusion beat generated by two impulses entering ventricle from different foci

Nursing/Medical Intervention

- Detect and document dysrhythmia; consider the circumstances in which it occurs
- Document frequency of the premature beats and any patterns of occurrence
- Evaluate sensorium, skin color/temperature
- Monitor hemodynamic parameters
- Monitor serum electrolytes
- Treat underlying cause
- Lidocaine (bolus/infusion)
- Procainamide

Ventricular escape complexes *should not* be suppressed.

Ventricular Tachycardia (VT)

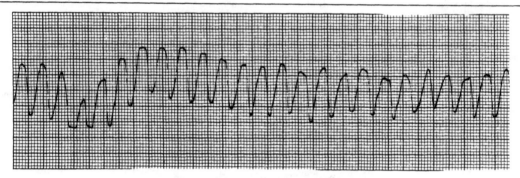

Figure 1.34   Ventricular Tachycardia

Etiology

- Acute MI
- Ischemic heart disease
- Aneurysm
- Rheumatic heart disease
- Metabolic disturbances
- Mitral valve prolapse
- Aortic valve disease
- Cardiomyopathy
- Drug toxicity (Isuprel, digitalis, quinidine)
- Ventricular ectopy
- Anxiety

Characteristics

- Rate: 100–250 BPM
- Rhythm: usually regular; may be slightly irregular
- P waves: not usually present
- QRS: ≥0.12 sec; may be uniform or polymorphic

Nursing/Medical Intervention

- Detect and document dysrhythmia, as it is potentially life-threatening
- Monitor hemodynamic parameters
- Assess sensorium, blood pressure, and peripheral pulses
- Evaluate signs/symptoms of diminished cardiac output
- Monitor serum electrolytes
- If pulseless, start CPR and deliver countershock

Refer to ACLS algorithm (Fig. 1.39).

- With pulse

Refer to ACLS algorithm (Fig. 1.44).

Ventricular Fibrillation[†]

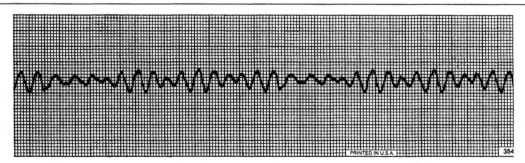

Figure 1.35   Ventricular Fibrillation

Etiology
- MI
- CAD
- Ischemia/reperfusion
- Electrolyte imbalance
- Metabolic acidosis
- Hypothermia
- Drugs (digitalis, quinidine, procainamide, cocaine)
- Ventricular tachycardia
- Electrocution

Characteristics
- Rate: extremely rapid
- Rhythm: chaotic
- P waves: none; PR not discernible
- QRS: wide, undifferentiated

Nursing/Medical Intervention
- Detect and document dysrhythmia
- Assess for signs/symptoms of diminished tissue perfusion
- If dysrhythmia verified, start CPR
- Asynchronous countershock
- Lidocaine
- Procainamide

Refer to ACLS algorithm (Fig. 1.40).

[†]Primary: sudden onset without hypotension or cardiac failure; secondary: terminal rhythm with circulatory failure.

Torsade de Pointes (Polymorphic VT)

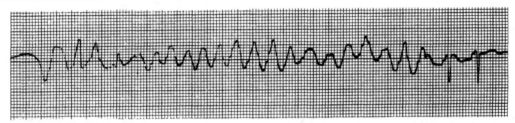

Figure 1.36 Torsades de Pointes

Etiology
- R on T ventricular extrasystole
- Prolonged QT interval
- Electrolyte imbalances
- Subarachnoid hemorrhage
- Class I antiarrhythmics

Characteristics
- Rate: may be >250 BPM
- Rhythm: irregular
- P waves: not identifiable
- QRS: wide; axis changes constantly producing "twisting" of points around the isoelectric axis

Nursing/Medical Intervention
- Identify dysrhythmia
- If patient unconscious, administer a precordial thump, electrical countershock, and CPR
- Treat underlying disorder (avoiding class 1a antiarrhythmic drugs)
- Magnesium sulfate
- Implantable defibrillator
- Ablative therapy

Ventricular Asystole

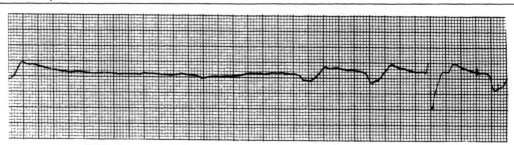

Figure 1.37   Ventricular Asystole

Etiology
- Acute respiratory failure
- MI
- Ischemia
- Valvular disease
- Hyperkalemia
- Ruptured ventricular aneurysm
- Enhanced vagal tone

Characteristics
- Rate: atrial—any; ventricular—none
- Rhythm: atrial—any; ventricular—none
- P waves: not present, normal or abnormal; no PR interval
- QRS: not visible

Loss of consciousness, peripheral pulses, blood pressure, and respirations, possibly seizures and death.

Nursing/Medical Intervention
- Detect and document pulselessness, apnea, and loss of consciousness
- Confirm asystole in two leads
- CPR
- Endoctracheal intubation
- Transvenous pacing
- Treat underlying cause

Refer to ACLS algorithm (Fig. 1.42).

Pulseless Electrical Activity (PEA)

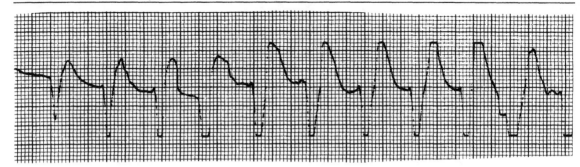

Figure 1.38   Pulseless Electrical Activity

Etiology
- Lack of heart muscle response to electrical stimulus
- Severe hypovolemia
- Pump failure
- Tension pneumothorax
- Cardiac tamponade
- PE
- Massive MI
- Hypoxemia/acidosis

Characteristics
- Heart fails to contract in the presence of a rhythm normally expected to produce a pulse

Nursing/Medical Intervention
- Document pulselessness, apnea and unresponsiveness
- Monitor ECG pattern normally expected to initiate a pulse
- Evaluate signs of circulatory collapse
- Monitor hemodynamic parameters
- CPR
- Endotracheal intubation
- Epinephrine
- Isuprel
- Treat underlying cause

Refer to ACLS algorithm (Fig. 1.41).

ACLS ALGORITHMS

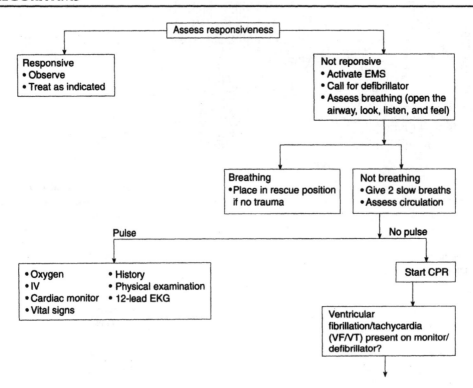

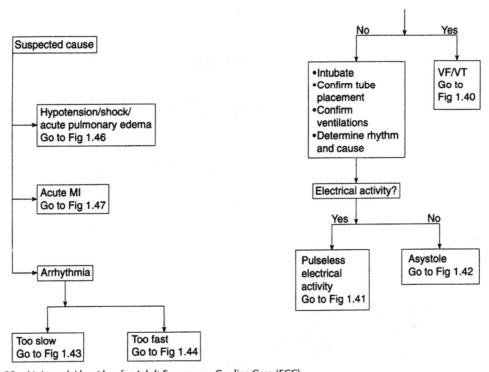

Figure 1.39 Universal Algorithm for Adult Emergency Cardiac Care (ECC)
Reproduced with permission. JAMA, October 28, 1992—Vol 268, No 16, p 2216. Copyright American Medical Association.

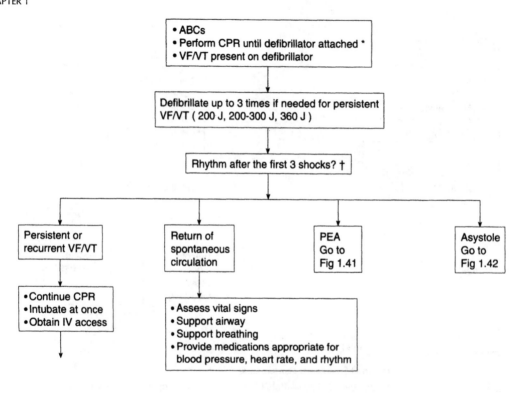

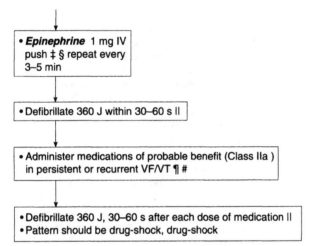

Figure 1.40 Algorithm for Ventricular Fibrillation and Pulseless Ventricular Tachycardia (VF/VT)

Reproduced with permission. JAMA, October 28, 1992—Vol 268, No 16, p 2217. Copyright American Medical Association.

Class I: definitely helpful

Class IIa: acceptable, probably helpful

Class IIb: acceptable, possibly helpful

Class III: not indicated, may be harmful

*Precordial thump is a Class IIb action in witnessed arrest, no pulse, and no defibrillator immediately available.

†Hypothermic cardiac arrest is treated differently after this point.

‡The recommended dose of *epinephrine* is 1 mg IV push every 3–5 min.

If this approach fails, several Class IIb dosing regimens can be considered:

- Intermediate: *epinephrine* 2–5 mg IV push, every 3–5 min
- Escalating: *epinephrine* 1 mg–3 mg–5 mg IV push (3 min apart)
- High: *epinephrine* 0.1 mg/kg IV push, every 3–5 min

§*Sodium bicarbonate* (1 mEq/kg) is Class I if patient has known preexisting hyperkalemia

‖Multiple sequenced shocks (200 J, 200–300 J, 360 J) are acceptable here (Class I), especially when medications are delayed.

¶ • *Lidocaine* 1.5 mg/kg IV push. Repeat in 3–5 min to total loading dose of 3 mg/kg; then use
- *Bretylium* 5 mg/kg IV push. Repeat in 5 min at 10 mg/kg
- *Magnesium sulfate* 1–2 g IV in torsades de pointes or suspected hypomagnesemic state or severe refractory VF
- *Procainamide* 30 mg/min in refractory VF (maximum total 17 mg/kg)

\# *Sodium bicarbonate* (1 mEq/kg IV):

Class IIa
- if known preexisting bicarbonate-responsive acidosis
- if overdose with tricyclic antidepressants
- to alkalinize the urine in drug overdoses

Class IIb
- if intubated and continued long arrest interval
- upon return of spontaneous circulation after long arrest interval

Class III
- hypoxic lactic acidosis

PEA includes:
- Electromechanical dissociation (EMD)
- Pseudo-EMD
- Idioventricular rhythms
- Ventricular escape rhythms
- Bradyasystolic rhythms
- Postdefibrillation idioventricular rhythms

- Continue CPR
- Intubate at once
- Obtain IV access
- Assess blood flow using Doppler ultrasound

Consider possible causes
(Parentheses = possible therapies and treatments)
- Hypovolemia (volume infusion)
- Hypoxia (ventilation)
- Cardiac tamponade (pericardiocentesis)
- Tension pneumothorax (needle decompression)
- Hypothermia
- Massive pulmonary embolism (surgery, *thrombolytics*)
- Drug overdoses such as tricyclics, digitalis, ß - blockers, calcium channel blockers
- Hyperkalemia *
- Acidosis †
- Massive acute myocardial infarction (go to Fig 1.47)

- *Epinephrine* 1 mg IV push, * ‡ repeat every 3–5 min

- If absolute bradycardia (< 60 beats/min) or relative bradycardia, give *atropine* 1 mg IV
- Repeat every 3–5 min up to a total of 0.04 mg/kg §

Figure 1.41 Algorithm for Pulseless Electrical Activity (PEA)—Electromechanical Dissociation (EMD)
Reproduced with permission. JAMA, October 28, 1992—Vol 268, No 16, p 2219. Copyright American Medical Association.

Class I: definitely helpful

Class IIa: acceptable, probably helpful

Class IIb: acceptable, possibly helpful

Class III: not indicated, may be harmful

Sodium bicarbonate 1 mEq/kg is Class I if patient has known preexisting hyperkalemia

†*Sodium bicarbonate* 1 mEq/kg:

    Class IIa

- if known preexisting bicarbonate-responsive acidosis
- if overdose with tricyclic antidepressants
- to alkalinize the urine in drug overdoses Class IIb
- if intubated and continued long arrest interval
- upon return of spontaneous circulation after long arrest interval

    Class III

- hypoxic lactic acidosis

‡The recommended dose of *epinephrine* is 1 mg IV push every 3–5 min. If this approach fails, several Class IIb dosing regimens can be considered.

- Intermediate: *epinephrine* 2–5 mg IV push, every 3–5 min
- Escalating: *epinephrine* 1 mg–3 mg–5 mg IV push (3 min apart)
- High: *epinephrine* 0.1 mg/kg IV push, every 3–5 min

§Shorter *atropine* dosing intervals are possibly helpful in cardiac arrest (Class IIb).

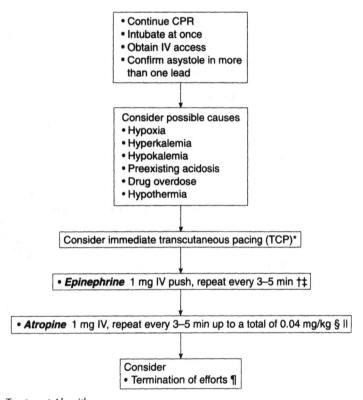

Figure 1.42 Asystole Treatment Algorithm

Reproduced with permission. JAMA, October 28, 1992—Vol 268, No 16, p 2220. Copyright American Medical Association.

Class I: definitely helpful

Class IIa: acceptable, probably helpful

Class IIb: acceptable, possibly helpful

Class III: not indicated, may be harmful

*TCP is a Class IIb intervention. Lack of success may be due to delays in pacing. To be effective TCP must be performed early, simultaneously with drugs. Evidence does not support routine use of TCP for asystole.

†The recommended dose of *epinephrine* is 1 mg IV push every 3–5 min. If this approach fails, several Class IIb dosing regimens can be considered:
- Intermediate: *epinephrine* 2–5 mg IV push, every 3–5 min
- Escalating: *epinephrine* 1 mg–3 mg–5 mg IV push (3 min apart)
- High: *epinephrine* 0.1 mg/kg IV push, every 3–5 min

§Shorter *atropine* dosing intervals are Class IIb in asystolic arrest

‡*Sodium bicarbonate* 1 mEq/kg is Class I if patient has known preexisting hyperkalemia

‖*Sodium bicarbonate* 1 mEq/kg:
  Class IIa
- if known preexisting bicarbonate-responsive acidosis
- if overdose with tricyclic antidepressants
- to alkalinize the urine in drug overdoses

  Class IIb
- if intubated and continued long arrest interval
- upon return of spontaneous circulation after long arrest interval

  Class III
- hypoxic lactic acidosis

¶ If patient remains in asystole or other agonal rhythms after successful intubation and initial medications and no reversible causes are identified, consider termination of resuscitative efforts by a physician. Consider interval since arrest.

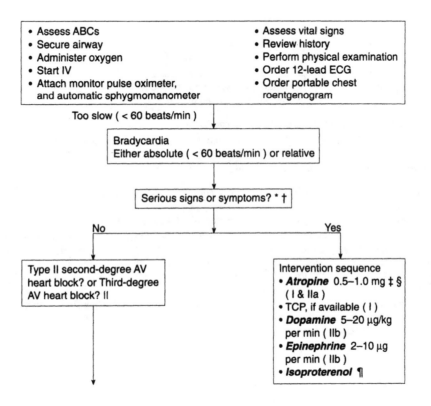

- Assess ABCs
- Secure airway
- Administer oxygen
- Start IV
- Attach monitor pulse oximeter,
  and automatic sphygmomanometer

- Assess vital signs
- Review history
- Perform physical examination
- Order 12-lead ECG
- Order portable chest
  roentgenogram

Too slow (< 60 beats/min)

Bradycardia
Either absolute (< 60 beats/min) or relative

Serious signs or symptoms? * †

No

Type II second-degree AV
heart block? or Third-degree
AV heart block? II

Yes

Intervention sequence
- *Atropine* 0.5–1.0 mg ‡ §
  (I & IIa)
- TCP, if available (I)
- *Dopamine* 5–20 μg/kg
  per min (IIb)
- *Epinephrine* 2–10 μg
  per min (IIb)
- *Isoproterenol* ¶

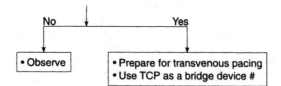

Figure 1.43   Bradycardia Algorithm (with the patient not in cardiac arrest)

Reproduced with permission. JAMA, October 28, 1992—Vol 268, No 16, p 2221. Copyright American Medical Association.

*Serious signs or symptoms must be related to the slow rate
Clinical manifestations include:
  symptoms (chest pain, shortness of breath, decreased level of consciousness) and signs (low BP, shock, pulmonary congestion, CHF, acute MI).

†Do not delay TCP while awaiting IV access or for atropine to take effect if patient is symptomatic

‡Denervated transplanted hearts will not respond to *atropine.* Go at once to pacing, *catecholamine* infusion, or both.

§*Atropine* should be given in repeat doses in 3–5 min up to total of 0.04 mg/kg. Consider shorter dosing intervals in severe
  clinical conditions. It has been suggested that atropine should be used with caution in atrioventricular (AV) block at the
  His-Purkinje level (type II AV block and new third-degree block with wide QRS complexes) (Class IIb).

‖Never treat third-degree heart block plus ventricular escape beats with *lidocaine.*

¶ *Isoproterenol* should be used, if at all, with extreme caution. At low doses it is Class IIb (possibly helpful); at higher doses it
  is Class III (harmful).

#Verify patient tolerance and mechanical capture. Use analgesia and sedation as needed.

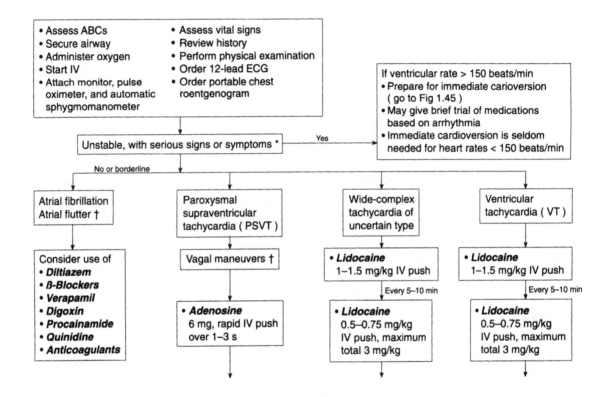

- Assess ABCs
- Secure airway
- Administer oxygen
- Start IV
- Attach monitor, pulse oximeter, and automatic sphygmomanometer

- Assess vital signs
- Review history
- Perform physical examination
- Order 12-lead ECG
- Order portable chest roentgenogram

If ventricular rate > 150 beats/min
- Prepare for immediate carioversion (go to Fig 1.45)
- May give brief trial of medications based on arrhythmia
- Immediate cardioversion is seldom needed for heart rates < 150 beats/min

Unstable, with serious signs or symptoms * → Yes

No or borderline

Atrial fibrillation Atrial flutter †

Paroxysmal supraventricular tachycardia (PSVT)

Wide-complex tachycardia of uncertain type

Ventricular tachycardia (VT)

Consider use of
- *Diltiazem*
- *ß-Blockers*
- *Verapamil*
- *Digoxin*
- *Procainamide*
- *Quinidine*
- *Anticoagulants*

Vagal maneuvers †

- *Lidocaine*
1–1.5 mg/kg IV push

- *Lidocaine*
1–1.5 mg/kg IV push

Every 5–10 min

- *Adenosine*
6 mg, rapid IV push over 1–3 s

- *Lidocaine*
0.5–0.75 mg/kg IV push, maximum total 3 mg/kg

Every 5–10 min

- *Lidocaine*
0.5–0.75 mg/kg IV push, maximum total 3 mg/kg

65

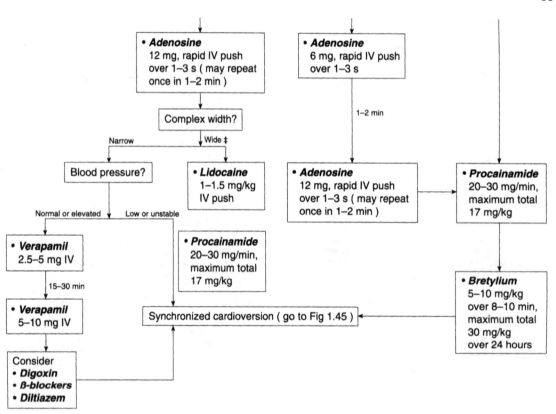

• **Adenosine**
12 mg, rapid IV push
over 1–3 s (may repeat
once in 1–2 min)

↓

Complex width?

Narrow ←   → Wide ‡

Blood pressure?

• **Lidocaine**
1–1.5 mg/kg
IV push

Normal or elevated   Low or unstable

• **Verapamil**
2.5–5 mg IV

↓ 15–30 min

• **Verapamil**
5–10 mg IV

Consider
• **Digoxin**
• **ß-blockers**
• **Diltiazem**

• **Procainamide**
20–30 mg/min,
maximum total
17 mg/kg

Synchronized cardioversion (go to Fig 1.45)

• **Adenosine**
6 mg, rapid IV push
over 1–3 s

1–2 min

• **Adenosine**
12 mg, rapid IV push
over 1–3 s (may repeat
once in 1–2 min)

• **Procainamide**
20–30 mg/min,
maximum total
17 mg/kg

• **Bretylium**
5–10 mg/kg
over 8–10 min,
maximum total
30 mg/kg
over 24 hours

Figure 1.44   Tachycardia Algorithm

Reproduced with permission. JAMA, October 28, 1992—Vol 268, No 16, p 2223. Copyright American Medical Association.

*Unstable condition must be related to the tachycardia. Signs and symptoms may include chest pain, shortness of breath, decreased level of consciousness, low blood pressure (BP), shock, pulmonary congestion, congestive heart failure, acute myocardial infarction.

†Carotid sinus pressure is contraindicated in patients with carotid bruits; avoid ice water immersion in patients with ischemic heart disease.

‡If the wide-complex tachycardia is known with certainty to be PSVT and BP is normal/elevated, sequence can include *verapamil.*

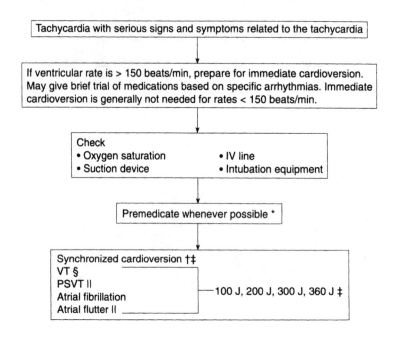

Tachycardia with serious signs and symptoms related to the tachycardia

If ventricular rate is > 150 beats/min, prepare for immediate cardioversion. May give brief trial of medications based on specific arrhythmias. Immediate cardioversion is generally not needed for rates < 150 beats/min.

Check
- Oxygen saturation
- Suction device
- IV line
- Intubation equipment

Premedicate whenever possible *

Synchronized cardioversion †‡
VT §
PSVT ‖
Atrial fibrillation
Atrial flutter ‖ ——————— 100 J, 200 J, 300 J, 360 J ‡

Figure 1.45   Electrical Cardioversion Algorithm (with the patient not in cardiac arrest)

Reproduced with permission. JAMA, October 28, 1992—Vol 268, No 16, p 2224. Copyright American Medical Association.

*Effective regimens have included a sedative (e.g., *diazepam, midazolam, barbiturates, etomidate, ketamine, methohexital*) with or without an analgesic agent (e.g., *fentanyl, morphine, meperidine*). Many experts recommend anesthesia if service is readily available.

†Note possible need to resynchronize after each cardioversion.

‡If delays in synchronization occur and clinical conditions are critical, go to immediate unsynchronized shocks.

§Treat polymorphic VT (irregular form and rate) like VF: 200 J, 200–300 J, 360 J.

∥PSVT and atrial flutter often respond to lower energy levels (start with 50 J).

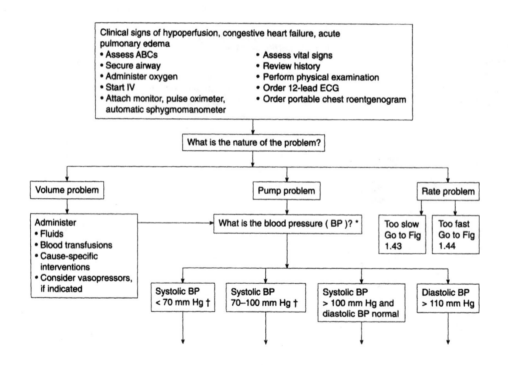

Clinical signs of hypoperfusion, congestive heart failure, acute
pulmonary edema
- Assess ABCs   • Assess vital signs
- Secure airway   • Review history
- Administer oxygen   • Perform physical examination
- Start IV   • Order 12-lead ECG
- Attach monitor, pulse oximeter,   • Order portable chest roentgenogram
  automatic sphygmomanometer

What is the nature of the problem?

Volume problem   Pump problem   Rate problem

Administer   What is the blood pressure (BP)? *   Too slow   Too fast
- Fluids   Go to Fig   Go to Fig
- Blood transfusions   1.43   1.44
- Cause-specific
  interventions
- Consider vasopressors,
  if indicated

Systolic BP   Systolic BP   Systolic BP   Diastolic BP
< 70 mm Hg †   70–100 mm Hg †   > 100 mm Hg and   > 110 mm Hg
                                          diastolic BP normal

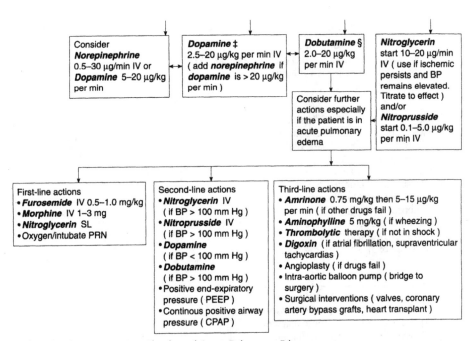

Figure 1.46 Algorithm for Hypotension, Shock, and Acute Pulmonary Edema

Reproduced with permission. JAMA, October 28, 1992—Vol 268, No 16, p 2227. Copyright American Medical Association.

*Base management after this point on invasive hemodynamic monitoring if possible.
†Fluid bolus of 250–500 mL normal saline should be tried. If no response, consider sympathomimetics.
‡Move to *dopamine* and stop *norepinephrine* when BP improves.
§Add *dopamine* when BP improves. Avoid *dobutamine* when systolic BP < 100 Hg.

```
┌─────────────────────────────────────────────────────┐
│                     Community                        │
│ • Community emphasis on " call first/call fast, call 911 " │
│ • National Heart Attack Alert Program                │
└─────────────────────────────────────────────────────┘
                          │
                          ▼
┌─────────────────────────────────────────────────────┐
│                    EMS System                        │
│ EMS system approach that should address              │
│ • Oxygen-IV-cardiac monitor-vital signs              │
│ • Nitroglycerin                                      │
│ • Pain relief with narcotics                         │
│ • Notification of emergency department               │
│ • Rapid transport to emergency department            │
│ • Prehospital screening for thrombolytic therapy *   │
│ • 12-lead ECG, computer analysis, transmission to    │
│   emergency department                               │
│ • Initiation of thrombolytic therapy *               │
└─────────────────────────────────────────────────────┘
                          │
                          ▼
┌─────────────────────────────────┐        ┌──────────────────┐
│       Emergency Department       │        │ Time interval    │
│  "Door-to-drug" team protocol approach │   │ in emergency     │
│ • Rapid triage of patients with chest pain │ │ department       │
│ • Clinical decision maker established │     └──────────────────┘
│   ( emergency physician, cardiologist, │          │
│   or other )                     │               │
└─────────────────────────────────┘               │
                │                                  │
                ▼                                  ▼
```

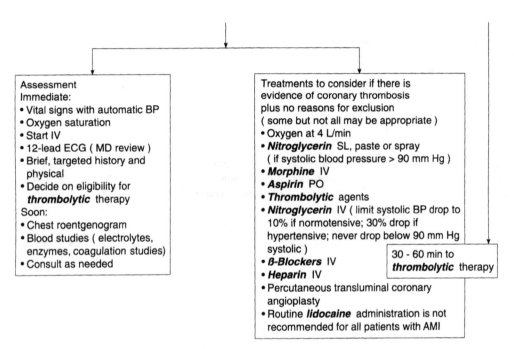

Figure 1.47 Acute Myocardial Infarction (AMI) Algorithm
Recommendations for early treatment of patients with chest pain and possible AMI.

Reproduced with permission. JAMA, October 28, 1992—Vol 268, No 16, p 2230. Copyright American Medical Association.

*Optional guidelines

COUNTERSHOCK

CARDIOVERSION
Synchronized/unsynchronized
Indications
- Atrial fibrillation
- Atrial flutter
- Supraventricular tachyarrhythmias
- Ventricular tachycardia

Indicators for unsynchronized cardioversion are hypotension, unconsciousness, or pulmonary edema. Unsynchronized cardioversion may be safer for rapid ventricular tachycardia, as the T wave may not be readily distinguished from the QRS. Nonsynchronized shock is less likely to fall on the T wave.

Preparation
- Informed consent (if patient is conscious and alert)
- If cardioversion is elective, and time permits, patient should take nothing by mouth for 8 hr prior to cardioversion
- Airway management
  - supplemental oxygen
  - assessment
  - acid–base balance (ABG analysis)
  - emergency equipment available
- Serum potassium (K^+) levels
  - correct as indicated
- Digoxin levels
  - cardioversion in the setting of digoxin toxicity can precipitate fatal ventricular arrhythmias
  - if necessary to cardiovert the digoxin toxic patient, use the lowest possible energy level (start at 10 J)
- Premedication/sedation
  - IV diazepam (Valium) 5–20 mg

– IV midazolam (Versed) 2.5–10 mg
– IV methohexital (Brevitol) 50–120 mg

In urgent situations or if the patient is obtunded, sedation may be omitted.

Technique
- Lubricate electrodes with gel
- Anterolateral paddle placement
  - place one paddle anteriorly over right upper sternal border
  - place other paddle laterally over left ventricular apex
- Anterior–posterior paddle replacement
  - place one paddle anteriorly, to left of lower sternal border
  - position other paddle posteriorly, at the angle of the left scapula
- Recommended energy levels
  - atrial fibrillation: 100 J initially, increasing in 100-J increments for each successive shock
  - atrial flutter: 10–25 J, depending on urgency of situation
  - PSVT: 75–100 J
  - ventricular tachycardia: 10–50 J initially, increasing to 100, 200, and 360 J as indicated

Various arrhythmias may occur as a result of cardioversion. Treatment of choice usually is pharmacological. If VF occurs: turn off the synchronizer circuit, charge the unit to 200 J, and defibrillate.

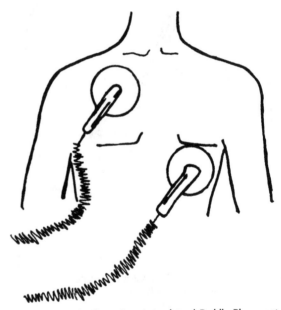

Figure 1.48A   Cardioversion: Anterolateral Paddle Placement

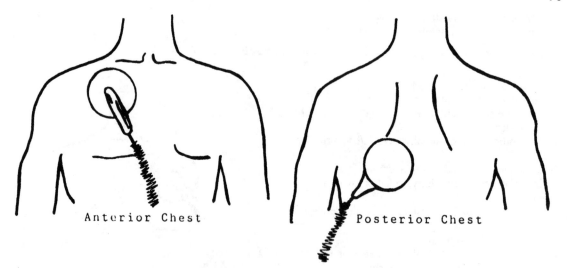

Figure 1.48B Cardioversion: Anterior–Posterior Paddle Placement

DEFIBRILLATION
Indications
- Cardiac arrest/asystole (confirm asystole in two leads/differentiate from fine VF)
- Pulseless ventricular tachycardia
- Ventricular fibrillation

Preparation
- Airway management; use supplemental oxygen
- Establish IV

Technique
- Lubricate electrodes well with gel
- Do not allow gel or paste to become continuous between the paddle sites or to reach the paddle handle, this may result in arcing and burns
- Anterolateral paddle placement
  - place one paddle anteriorly over right upper sternal border
  - place other paddle laterally over left ventricular apex
- Recommended energy levels
  - 200 J initially
  - 300 and 360 J subsequently if pulse does not return

Permanent Pacemaker
- Place defibrillation paddles or electrodes as far away from pulse generator as possible
- Anteriolateral paddle placement delivers defibrillation energy in same direction as pacemaker sensing vector and may damage pulse generator
- Anterior–posterior paddle position reduces potential for pacemaker damage
- Use lowest clinically appropriate energy
- Following defibrillation, pulse generator performance should be verified

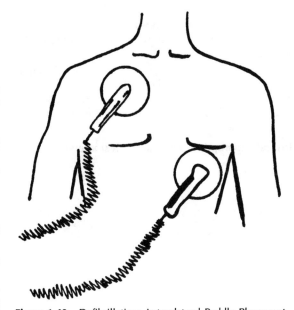

Figure 1.49 Defibrillation: Anterolateral Paddle Placement

CARDIAC EVALUATION AND MANAGEMENT

77

Temporary Transvenous Pacemaker
- Turn off or disconnect pulse generator prior to defibrillation

Implantable Defibrillator
- If ventricular tachycardia or ventricular fibrillation persists beyond functional capacity of the AICD, an external countershock should be delivered
- Unsuccessful external defibrillation may result from paddle placement over the AICD patch electrodes. These electrodes may insulate heart muscle from defibrillation shocks. Change placement of paddle electrodes and defibrillate

Institute appropriate pharmacological interventions

PACEMAKERS

Function
- Stimulates the heart to contract via myocardial cell depolarization

Components
- Pulse generator
  - consists of a power source (battery) and electronic circuitry
  - may have a sensing mechanism, which interprets information about patient's intrinsic rhythm
  - may be external or implanted
- Pacing leads
  - may be unipolar or bipolar
  - both electrodes sense patient's spontaneous cardiac activity; negative (cathode) lead delivers the electrical impulse
  - electrode must have direct contact with myocardium to elicit depolarization and contraction
  - permanent pacemaker leads include:
    - tined atrial J lead (seals in the atrial appendage)
    - active fixation (screw-in) lead
    - tined lead
    - finned lead
    - steroid tip (delivers steroid dosage to myocardium) to reduce fibrotic growth
- Bridging cable
  - an extension wire that allows external pacemaker to be secured away from insertion site for patient comfort and safety

Figure 1.50 Implanted Pacemakers: The Synergyst™ II Dual-Chamber Rate-Responsive Pacemaker; the Legend™ Single-Chamber Rate-Responsive Pacemaker; and the Minix™ Single-Chamber Pacemaker (about the size of a large coin)

Shown (Left to Right) with the pulse generators are the Cap-Sure® and Target Tip® Bipolar Pacing Leads and the Three Myocardial Leads. The CapSure® Lead releases a steroid that facilitates optimum receptivity of the pacing impulse by the heart muscle.

Used with permission from Medtronic, Inc.

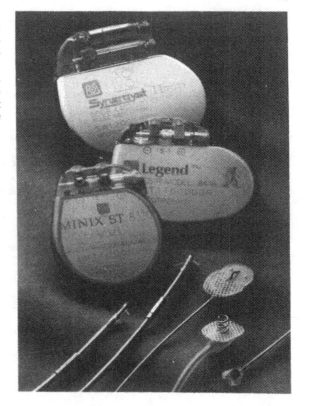

TEMPORARY PACING

Indications
- Immediate need for pacing
  - complete heart block with slow ventricular response
  - symptomatic sinus bradycardia, prolonged sinus pauses, asystole
  - anterior MI with complete heart block
  - inferior MI with complete heart block, poorly tolerated rates, CHF, hypotension, ventricular arrhythmias
  - Mobitz type II
  - new bifascicular block
  - torsade de pointes induced by drugs or bradycardia
  - atrial flutter
  - recurrent, sustained ventricular tachycardia
  - malfunction of an implanted permanent pacemaker
  - prophylactically; cardiac catheterization, cardioversion, angioplasty

Contraindications
- Systemic sepsis

Temporary pacing usually is an emergency procedure; there are no *absolute* contraindications.

Risks
- Complications related to vascular access
  - pneumothorax
  - hemothorax
  - thrombophlebitis
- Catheter manipulation
  - ventricular fibrillation or flutter

Acute MI Increases Risk
- Right ventricular perforation
  - pericardial friction rub
  - cardiac tamponade

Insertion
- Transthoracic
  - pacing wire placed into right ventricular myocardium by way of an introducer through chest wall
  - risks of this procedure include hemorrhage, coronary artery injury with pericardial tamponade
- Transvenous (endocardial pacing)
  - pacing wire threaded through a selected vein into right atrium or ventricle
    - internal jugular: advantages include a direct route to right side of heart, may be accomplished without fluoroscopy, catheter is stable, rapid insertion time. Disadvantages include risk of carotid artery perforation, some risk of hemo/pneumothorax, may be dislodged with movement of head.
    - subclavian vein: advantages include easy accessibility, stability, rapid insertion time. Disadvantages are risk of subclavian artery perforation, hemo/pneumothorax
    - basilic vein: advantages include easy accessibility, reduced risk of hemo/pneumothorax. Disadvantages involve catheter instability, increased risk of cardiac perforation, necessity of fluoroscopy
    - femoral vein: advantages include easy access to right heart using fluoroscopy, rapid insertion time. Disadvantages involve risk of dislodgment by leg movement, high risk of thrombophlebitis

Pertinent Points
- Defibrillatory shocks may damage a temporary pacemaker; after defibrillation, carefully test the pacemaker
- Temporary pacemaker may fail at hyperbaric conditions of 50 to 60 psi
- Lead terminal of the temporary pacemaker is outside patient's body, constituting an electrocution hazard

Measuring Stimulation Thresholds[†]
- With the pacemaker turned *OFF*, set the *OUTPUT* control at 5 mA
- Set the *RATE* control at least 10 ppm (pulses per minute) above the patient's intrinsic rate
- Set the sensitivity control halfway between 1.5 mV and 3 mV
- Connect the pacemaker to the patient and turn the pacemaker *ON*
- Verify (on ECG) 1:1 capture of the heart by a pacing stimulus
- Gradually decrease the output current until 1:1 capture is lost
- Gradually increase the output current to find the amplitude at which capture is regained—the stimulation threshold
- Reset the *OUTPUT* control at 5 mA or a setting that is at least double the stimulation threshold

Measuring Sensitivity Thresholds[†]
- Set the *SENSITIVITY* control halfway between 1.5 mV and 3 mV
- Set the *RATE* control at least 10 ppm below the patient's intrinsic rate
- Set the *OUTPUT* control at 5 mA
- The pacemaker should stop pacing (see ECG) and the sense indicator start flashing as the unit senses naturally occurring R waves
- Gradually turn the *SENSITIVITY* control counterclockwise until the pacemaker begins firing pacing stimuli and the *PACE* indicator begins flashing—the sensitivity threshold
- Reset the *SENSITIVITY* control 2 to 3 times more sensitive than the threshold level

Typical Acceptable Thresholds[†]

Stimulation Thresholds[‡] (maximum values)

Ventricular	1.0 mA
Atrial	2.0 mA

Sensitivity Threshold (minimum R wave value)

Ventricular	3.0 mV or more

[†]Used with permission from Medtronic, Inc.

[‡]May vary according to lead system used.

Troubleshooting[†]

Situation	*Probable Cause*	*Correct Approach*
Loss of pacemaker artifact	Pacemaker too sensitive	Reduce sensitivity (turn sensitivity dial toward asynchronous or higher mV value)
	Battery depletion	Change battery
	Loose, broken, or disconnected wires	Change external pacemaker
	Short circuit of wire	Repair or replace pacing catheter or ground wire
Failure to capture without loss of pacing	Catheter malposition	Increase output; reposition patient; reposition catheter
	Battery depletion	Change battery
	Electronic insulation break	Change external pacemaker
	Output setting too low	Increase output; repair insulation; change catheter
Rate malfunction	Faulty external pacemaker	Change external pacemaker
Loss of proper sensing	Catheter malposition	Reposition catheter
	Pacemaker not sensitive enough	Increase sensitivity (turn dial toward lower mV value)
	Faulty external pacemaker	Change external pacemaker
	Electrical interference caused reversion to asynchronous	Eliminate interference

Oversensing	Pacemaker too sensitive	Decrease sensitivity (turn sensitivity dial toward asynchronous or higher mV value)
	Electrical interference	Eliminate interference; change external pacemaker
Pacemaker-induced arrhythmias	Output setting too high	Decrease output
	Electrical interference	Eliminate interference
	Altered threshold	Change mode or setting
		Appropriate drugs
Stimulation of chest wall or diaphragm	Output too high	Reduce output
	Perforation	Change patient's position; reposition catheter

Disclaimer: The acceptable thresholds and typical settings previously stated may vary according to the individual patient's condition, physician's recommended procedure, and standard hospital procedure.

†Used with permission from Medtronic, Inc.

‡May vary according to lead system used.

Temporary Pacemaker Code—Three-Letter NBG Pacemaker Code (1987)

Chamber Paced	Chamber Sensed	Sensed Response
V–Ventricle	V–Ventricle	T–Triggers pacing
A–Atrium	A–Atrium	I–Inhibits pacing
D–Dual (A + V)	D–Dual (A + V)	D–Dual
O–None	O–None	O–None

Used with permission from Medtronic, Inc.

PERMANENT PACING
Indications
- Symptomatic bradyarrhythmias
- Severe asymptomatic bradyarrhythmias
- Acquired AV block
- Complete (intranodal) heart block
- Symptomatic Mobitz I
- Mobitz II
- Atrial flutter or fibrillation with slow ventricular response
- Sick sinus syndrome
- Tachybrady syndrome

Contraindications
- Few other than risks

Risks
- Catheter dislodgment
- Lead fracture
- Pacemaker system failure
- Erosion of pulse generator
- Pacemaker induced tachycardia
- Infection
- Cardiac perforation with tamponade
- Thrombosis of superior vena cava or right atrium

Insertion
- Venous access
  - cephalic vein
    - in a small segment of the population, cephalic vein may be absent or rudimentary
  - subclavian vein
    - in dual chamber pacing, cephalic vein is sufficient only for ventricular lead; subclavian vein may be used for atrial lead
  - internal/external jugular
    - may be used if cephalic vein is not available

Programmability
- Escape rate
  - interval between the last sensed beat and the following pacemaker beat

- Hysteresis
  - allows pacemaker to *inhibit* at a level below the set paced level to allow for reduced rate when patient is at rest or asleep
  - a factor of energy storage
  - no hysteresis level on a rate responsive pacemaker
- Refractory period
  - period during which a pulse generator is unresponsive to input signals

Pertinent Points
- A 10% decrease of the original set rate is an indicator for battery change
- A magnet placed over the pacemaker converts it to an asynchronous nonpacing mode (for diagnostic purposes)
- Surgical cautery may inhibit the unit or convert it to an asynchronous mode
- Pacemaker patients, particularly those with unipolar units, should avoid TENS unit.
- Defibrillators may cause damage to pacemaker circuitry; if defibrillation is imperative, place paddles as far from pulse generator as possible; after shock has been administered, pacemaker should be checked meticulously
- Exposures to diagnostic X-rays constitutes no problems for the pacemaker, but therapeutic radiation may cause the pulse generator to malfunction
- MRI may cause conversion to a fixed rate or false inhibition

NBG Pacemaker Code (1987)

I Chamber Paced	II Chamber Sensed	III Response to Sensing	IV Programmable Functions; Rate Modulation	V Antitachyarrhythmia Function(s)
V–ventricle	V–ventricle	T–triggers pacing	P–programmable rate and/or output	P–pacing (antitachyarrhythmia)
A–atrium	A–atrium	I–inhibits pacing	M–multiprogrammability of rate, output, sensitivity, etc.	S–shock
D–dual (A + V)	D–dual (A + V)	D–dual (T + I)	C–communicating functions (telemetry)	D–dual (P + S)
O–none	O–none	O–none	R–rate modulation	O–none
S*–A or V	S*–A or V		O–none	

*Used by manufacturers

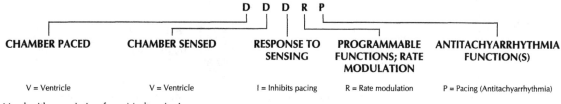

CHAMBER PACED	CHAMBER SENSED	RESPONSE TO SENSING	PROGRAMMABLE FUNCTIONS; RATE MODULATION	ANTITACHYARRHYTHMIA FUNCTION(S)
V = Ventricle	V = Ventricle	I = Inhibits pacing	R = Rate modulation	P = Pacing (Antitachyarrhythmia)

Used with permission from Medtronic, Inc.

Decision Algorithm for Selection of Cardiac Pacemakers

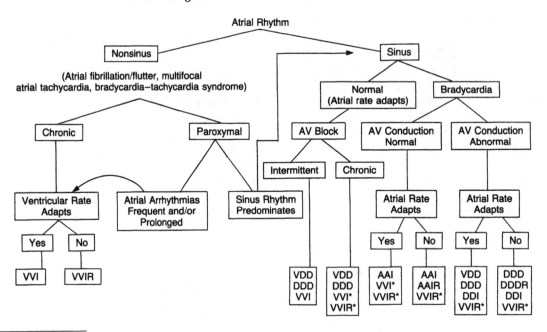

*Ventricular pacing indicated if atrial sensing and/or pacing is not possible, and if the patient is sedentary and elderly
Reprinted with permission from Satinder JS and Goldschlager N: Selecting the Best Cardiac Pacing System, *Choices in Cardiology*, 3(1):26, 1989.

NONINVASIVE PACING

Function
- Delivers electrical stimulus to the heart, resulting in cardiac depolarization and myocardial contraction
- During pacing, monitor patient constantly; adhere to usual protocol for emergency measures (airway management, CPR, drug therapy)

Indications
- Asystole
- Pulseless idioventricular rhythm
- Symptomatic bradycardia unresponsive to drug therapy
- Termination of tachyarrhythmias (atrial/ventricular)
- Transient conduction disturbances
- Stokes–Adams attacks associated with heart block
- Drug toxicity
- Implanted pacemaker failure/malfunction
- In situations where transvenous pacing would constitute a hazard to patient
  - artificial tricuspid valve
  - suppressed immune system with increased potential for infection
  - systemic infection
  - bleeding disorders
  - present or recent thrombolytic therapy

Contraindications
- Prolonged cardiac arrest
- Severe metabolic disorders
- Cardiac trauma
- EMD
- Extensive MI
- Extensive damage to cardiac conduction system

Components
- Pulse generator
  - delivers required current to heart
- Cables
  - connect pulse generator and electrodes
- Electrodes
  - adhesive pads placed on chest and back
- ECG monitor and defibrillator included in some newer models

Pacing Modes
- Asynchronous (fixed rate/nondemand)
  - delivers electrical stimulus at a selected rate
  - used less frequently than demand because of the danger involved in delivering a stimulus during heart's vulnerable period (R on T)
  - may be used for overdrive or underdrive pacing to terminate tachydysrhythmias
- Synchronous (demand)
  - delivers electrical stimulus only when needed
  - pulse generator senses heart's intrinsic QRS complexes
  - sensitivity adjusted by altering ECG size, gain, or sensitivity control
  - pacemaker inhibited when an intrinsic beat sensed
  - minimizes competition between patient's intrinsic rate and pacemaker

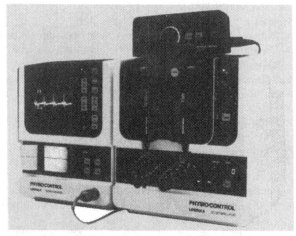

Figure 1.51 Noninvasive Pacemaker Consisting of an ECG Monitor, a Defibrillator, and a Pacemaker in a Single Device

Noninvasive Pacing—What You Should Know. Reprinted with permission of Physio-Control Corp., 1988.

Electrode Placement
- Electrode placement and polarity are important
  - may affect the pacing current threshold and patient comfort
  - preferred placement is anterior–posterior position, with negative electrode placed on the left anterior chest between the xyphoid and the nipple line; positive electrode placed on the left posterior chest beneath the scapula, lateral to the spine; in women, negative electrode placed just below the left breast
  - if anterior–posterior placement is impossible, use anterior–anterior; negative electrode placed on the left chest midaxilla at the 4th ICS; positive electrode placed on the anterior right chest, subclavicular; anterior–anterior placement is less desirable—it causes pectoral muscle stimulation and interferes with defibrillator paddle placement

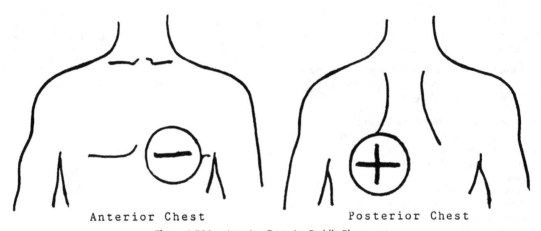

Anterior Chest   Posterior Chest

Figure 1.52A   Anterior–Posterior Paddle Placement

- Electrodes should be placed on clean dry skin
  - if chest hair constitutes a problem, clip it rather than shave it; shaving may leave small nicks in the skin, increasing patient discomfort during pacing
- When peeling the protector pack off the electrode back
  - handle the electrode carefully
  - do not contaminate adhesive border of electrode with gel; gel on adhesive border may compromise that area of electrode; patient's skin can be burned by displaced gel
  - press on the electrode adhesive area first
  - electrodes may be kept in place for 24 to 72 hours (validate with manufacturer)

While a noninvasive pacer is in the pacing mode, do not touch gelled area of electrode; a minor electrical shock hazard exists.

Patient Response to Noninvasive Pacing

- Both electrical and mechanical capture must occur if noninvasive pacing is to be of benefit
  - indicators of electrical capture are
    - a wide QRS
    - a tall, broad T wave
  - indicators of mechanical (ventricular) capture are
    - improved cardiac output
    - increase in B/P
    - palpable pulse
    - improvement of skin color/temperature

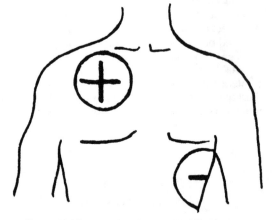

Figure 1.52B   Anterior–Anterior Paddle Placement

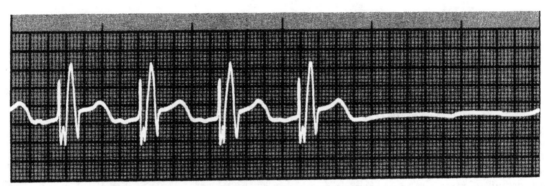

Figure 1.53 Example of Electrical Capture, Showing a Wide QRS and Tall T Wave
Noninvasive Pacing—What You Should Know. Reprinted with permission of Physio-Control Corp., 1988.

Electrical capture without mechanical capture can indicate that patient may not be viable (such as with expensive MI, prolonged cardiac arrest, etc.).

- Skeletal muscle contraction expected
  - does not indicate pacemaker capture
  - common subjective assessments verbalized
    - tap
    - thud
    - tingle
    - twitch
    - range from tolerable to intolerable

- To reduce discomfort of the conscious patient
  - reposition anterior (negative) electrode to the ECG V_6 position
  - reposition anterior (negative) electrode to the epigastric area

Placement results in a lower capture threshold, reducing discomfort.
  - in some instances sedation and/or analgesia may be indicated

Defibrillation During Noninvasive Pacing
- Defibrillate promptly if VF occurs
- May leave some noninvasive models on during defibrillation; others must be turned off (validate with manufacturer)
- Place defibrillation paddles in standard apex-sternum position
- Do not place defibrillation paddles on patient electrodes
- After defibrillation, remove any gel or moisture that may have accumulated on patient's chest or bed linens

CPR During Noninvasive Pacing
- CPR and noninvasive pacing may be performed simultaneously
- Be sure that the pacing electrodes firmly adhere to chest
- Occasionally, operator may feel slight tingling or muscle twitching in hands; if sensation is strong or painful, pacing and CPR should not be performed simultaneously

QUIK-COMBO™ DEFIBRILLATOR/MONITOR/ PACEMAKER ACCESSORY—PACING/ DEFIBRILLATION/SHOCK ADVISORY ADAPTER

This adapter adds automated external defibrillator (AED) features to the LIFEPAK 9 P defibrillator/monitor/ pacemaker. AED features identify shockable rhythms and cue basic life support (BLS) providers through the defibrillation process. With this adapter, the QUIK-COMBO™ electrode set can monitor ECG and deliver synchronized cardioversion, defibrillation, and noninvasive pacing therapy. The system analyzes ECG wavelengths, determines if a rhythm is shockable, and provides the operator with advisory messages (i.e., SHOCK ADVISED! PUSH CHARGE, or NO SHOCK ADVISED).

Indications
- Defibrillation
- Synchronized cardioversion
- Noninvasive pacing therapy
- ECG monitoring

Pertinent Points
- The QUIK-COMBO™ adapter or the QUIK-COMBO™ connector must be securely locked or ineffective energy delivery may result in intermittent operation and inability to perform the monitoring, defibrillation, or pacing functions

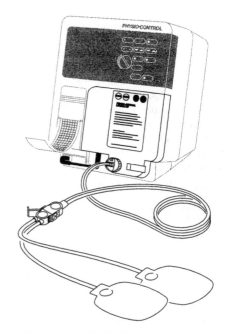

Figure 1.54 Installed QUIK-COMBO Adapter

Reprinted with permission of Physio-Control Corporation, January 1995.

- The QUIK-COMBO therapy cable must **NOT** be connected directly to the defibrillator—defibrillation and pacing therapy can be delivered only with the QUIK-COMBO adapter
- Do not connect standard paddles to the QUIK-COMBO adapter; connection of these paddles to the adapter renders the discharge button inoperative
- Only QUIK-COMBO electrodes can be used with the QUIK-COMBO therapy cable
- Do not place QUIK-COMBO electrodes in anterior–posterior position; the shock advisory system requires anterior–lateral placement
- Equipment that emits certain radio frequency signals may interfere with ECG signals, resulting in inaccurate rhythm analysis
- Make certain to securely attach the interconnect cable to the defibrillator before turning the power on; failure to do so may result in inability to deliver therapy

Not for use with pediatric patients

QUIK-COMBO™ Adapter Features

1 – ANALYZE: ECG rhythm analysis
2 – CHARGE: Initiates the defibrillator charge cycle (charge is available for 1 min before it is automatically removed)
3 – DISCHARGE BUTTONS: Discharge defibrillator. Buttons must be pressed simultaneously to deliver energy. Energy cannot be delivered unless device is fully charged to preselected level.
4 – CONNECTOR

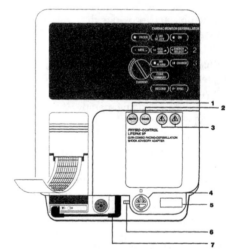

Figure 1.55   QUIK-COMBO Adapter Features

Reprinted with permission of Physio-Control Corporation, January 1995.

5 – TEST LOAD CONNECTOR: Performs defibrillation test using 200 J
6 – LOCK LEVER: Locks QUIK-COMBO adapter in place; up position is locked, down position unlocked
7 – INTERCONNECT CABLE: Connects pacing output from the device to QUIK-COMBO adapter

NOT SHOWN (DEFIB OUT): The DEFIBRILLATOR OUTPUT CONNECTOR (Connector site for use with black cable connectors, such as standard paddles, internal handles **with** discharge control, difibrillation adapter, and QUIK-COMBO adapter)

Installing and Removing the QUIK-COMBO™ Adapter
The QUIK-COMBO adapter fits in the paddle storage area of the LIFEPAK 9 P defibrillator. The standard paddles must be removed before installing this adapter.

Disconnecting Standard Paddles
1. Remove the paddles from the defibrillator paddle storage area
2. Rotate the connector locking ring (attached to the paddles) counterclockwise and turn until a positive stop is reached and connector arrows are aligned
3. Grasp the connector body and gently pull until the black connector separates from the DEFIB OUT connector on the defibrillator

Installing the QUIK-COMBO™ Adapter
1. Push the yellow locking lever down on the QUIK-COMBO adapter
2. Insert the top of the QUIK-COMBO adapter into the paddle storage area on the defibrillator, then push the bottom of the adapter into the DEFIB OUT connector (see Fig. 1.56)

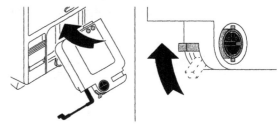

Figure 1.56 Installing the QUIK-COMBO Adapter and Locking in Place

Reprinted with permission of Physio-Control Corporation, January 1995.

3. Push the yellow locking lever **up** to lock adapter in place (see Fig. 1.56)
4. Insert the interconnect cable on the adapter firmly into the pacing output connector on the defibrillator (see Fig. 1.57). Do not twist the cable.

Removing the QUIK-COMBO™ Adapter

1. Make sure the QUIK-COMBO electrodes are disconnected from the QUIK-COMBO therapy cable
2. Unplug the interconnect cable on the adapter from the pacing output connector on the defibrillator
3. Push the yellow locking lever down to unlock the adapter
4. Lift the bottom of the adapter and pull out

When connecting the QUIK-COMBO therapy cable, connect accessory connections black to black and gray to gray.

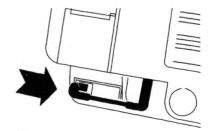

Figure 1.57   Plugging in the Interconnect Cable

Reprinted with permission of Physio-Control Corporation, January 1995.

Installing and removing the QUIK-COMBO™ Adapter information reprinted with permission of Physio-Control (11811 Willows Road Northeast, Redmond, WA 98073-9723), and Operating Instructions for LIFEPAK 9 P, January 1995.

Troubleshooting the QUIK-COMBO™ Adapter

Problem

No ECG trace or excessive noise on screen

Corrective Action

- Check
  - that the device is powered on
  - that LEAD SELECT is set to PADDLES
  - that the QUIK-COMBO adapter is fully seated and locked in place
  - that the QUIK-COMBO therapy cable is connected and locked to the adapter
  - that the QUIK-COMBO therapy cable is connected to the QUIK-COMBO electrodes
  - for poor skin preparation, poor electrode contact, or outdated or damaged QUIK-COMBO electrodes
  - for cable damage; replace if necessary
  - for motion or radio frequency interference source

Adapter controls will not activate

- Check
  - that the device is powered on
  - that the QUIK-COMBO adapter is fully seated and locked
  - that the QUIK-COMBO therapy cable is connected and locked to adapter
  - that charging is complete

Defibrillator will not discharge

- Check
  - that the device is powered on
  - that QUIK-COMBO adapter is fully seated and locked
  - that charging is complete

To ANALYZE: CONNECT DEFIB PADS
message appears

- Check
  - if the QUIK-COMBO electrodes are detached from patient
  - if the QUIK-COMBO therapy cable connector is detached from electrodes
  - if the QUIK-COMBO therapy cable is detached from the adapter

To ANALYZE: STOP MOTION and/or
MOTION DETECTED, CANNOT ANALYZE
message appears

- Stop all motion, do not touch patient; motion or other ECG signal interference may be preventing ECG rhythm analysis
  - Assess patient—patient may be conscious and breathing
  - Stop any patient contact
  - Stop moving cables or touching electrodes
  - Stop compression, ventilation and allow for completion of passive exhalation if resuscitation is in progress
  - Press firmly on and around the QUIK-COMBO electrodes to ensure adequate adhesion to patient; if poor adhesion persists, replace electrodes with a new pair

	– Eliminate exposure to excessive radio frequency interference by distancing the device from electrical sources such as high output radios, antennas, or electric blankets
	• Replace the QUIK-COMBO therapy cable if motion detected when the device is connected to a Physio-Control patient simulator and MOTION is not being activated. If the condition persists, call a qualified service technician.
	• Check the QUIK-COMBO therapy cable connector for wear. Perform periodic cable tests; if a cable fails the "cable shake" test, it must be replaced.
SERVICE ADAPTER message appears	• Remove the adapter from service. Call a qualified service technician.
CONNECT PACING LEADS message appears	• Check – that the device is powered on – if the interconnect cable is detached from the device – if the QUIK-COMBO adapter and QUIK-COMBO therapy cable are detached
	• Remove the adapter from service. Call a qualified service technician.

Troubleshooting the QUIK-COMBO™ adapter information reprinted with permission of Physio-Control, Redmond, WA, and Operating Instructions for LIFEPAK 9 P, January 1995.

COUNTERPULSATION: INTRA-AORTIC BALLOON PUMP (IABP)

Function
- Balloon inflation
  - augmentation of coronary blood flow
  - increase of coronary collateral circulation
  - augmentation of perfusion to aortic arch and systemic circulation
- Balloon deflation
  - reduction of left ventricular afterload
  - decreased myocardial oxygen consumption
  - enhanced cardiac output
  - reduces shunting/regurgitant blood flow in septal/valvular defects

Indications
- Acute MI
- Ventricular aneurysm
- Inability to wean from cardiopulmonary bypass
- Severe CHF
- Shock states (cardiac/noncardiac)
- Unstable angina refractory to maximal medical therapy
- PTCA complications/impending infarction

Contraindications
- Aortic aneurysm
- Aortic insufficiency
- Aortic wall abnormality
- Chronic end-stage heart disease
- Irreversible brain damage
- Severe bleeding diathesis

Use with caution in patients with peripheral vascular disease.

Components

- An elongated balloon mounted on a catheter placed in the descending thoracic aorta
- Catheter may consist of semiflexible tubing with a single gas lumen or a double lumen catheter with a hollow central lumen; both catheters are approximately 36 in long; balloon is mounted on the distal 10 in; inflation capacity of balloon is approximately 40 cc
- A console that controls balloon inflation and deflation, monitors ECG and arterial tracings, and provides hard-copy documentation
- A tank of carbon dioxide (CO_2) or helium gas used as the balloon inflation medium

Triggering (activation of inflation/deflation)

- Indicators
  - R wave of the ECG: inflation takes place in diastole; deflation just prior to systole
  - arterial wave: pump activated by upstroke of arterial wave; pulse pressure must be at least 20 mm Hg
  - intrinsic pump rate: pump may be set to inflate and deflate at a preset (intrinsic) heart rate

Balloon pumping will not effectively replace cardiac compressions during cardiopulmonary resuscitation. Counterpulsation should be discontinued during CPR. To prevent thrombus formation during CPR the balloon must be manually inflated and deflated. This is accomplished by rapidly inflating and deflating the balloon with a 20-cc syringe several times every 10 min with a volume of air equal to one-half the balloon volume.

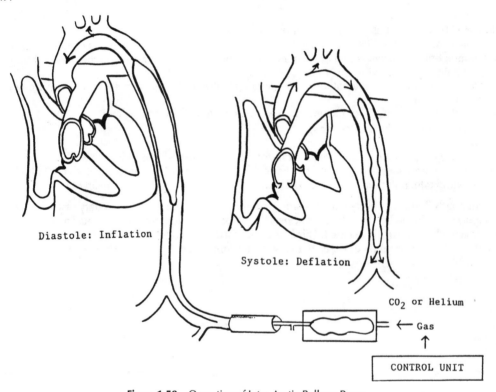

Diastole: Inflation

Systole: Deflation

CO_2 or Helium

← Gas

CONTROL UNIT

Figure 1.58   Operation of Intra-Aortic Balloon Pump

Figure 1.59 Intra-Aortic Balloon Pump

Reprinted with permission of Datascope Corp. (14 Phillips Parkway, Montvale, NJ 07645), 1995.

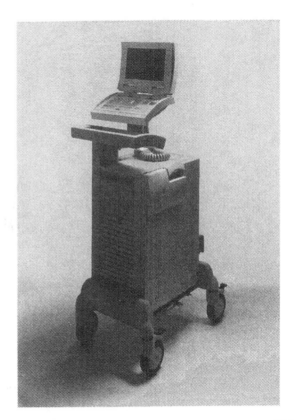

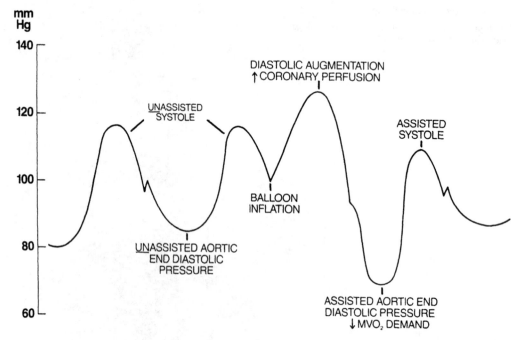

Figure 1.60   Variations in Arterial Waveform

Mechanics of Intra-Aortic Balloon Counterpulsation. Reprinted with permission of Datascope Corp. Clinical Education Services, 1989.

Timing (onset of balloon inflation/deflation)
- Indicator
  - arterial wave form: systole/diastole cannot be adequately identified from ECG
- Should be checked
  - at least every 2 hr
  - if cardiac index changes
  - when triggering mode is changed (1:1, 1:2, etc.)
  - development of arrhythmias
  - 20% change in heart rate (faster/slower)

If rhythms are rapid or grossly irregular, regular manual timing may be impossible; automatic timing is best used in these instances.

When a patient has a pacemaker, the pacing spikes act as the ECG trigger. With single-chamber atrial or dual chamber pacing, the atrial spikes may trigger premature balloon deflation and alter inflation timing.

Effects of Inappropriate Triggering/Timing

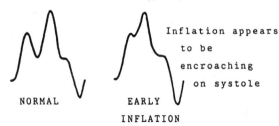

Figure 1.61   Early Inflation

Seminar for Intra-Aortic Balloon Pumping. Reprinted with permission of Datascope Corp. Clinical Educational Services, 1986.

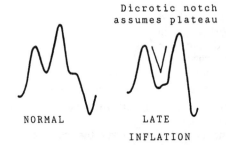

Figure 1.62   Late Inflation

Seminar for Intra-Aortic Balloon Pumping. Reprinted with permission of Datascope Corp. Clinical Educational Services, 1986.

Waveform begins above the dicrotic notch.

- Balloon inflates before aortic valve closes
- Increases work of left ventricle
- Increases pressure against which left ventricle must pump

Adjust timing; inflate later.

Augmented waveform is below the dicrotic notch.

- Balloon inflates in a partially filled aorta
- Deprives coronary arteries of adequate perfusion

Adjust timing; inflate earlier.

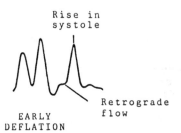

```
Rise in
systole
```

EARLY
DEFLATION

Retrograde
flow

Figure 1.63 Early Deflation

Seminar for Intra-Aortic Balloon Pumping. Reprinted with
permission of Datascope Corp. Clinical Educational Services,
1986.

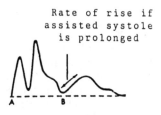

```
Rate of rise if
assisted systole
is prolonged
```

LATE DEFLATION

Figure 1.64 Late Deflation

Seminar for Intra-Aortic Balloon Pumping. Reprinted with
permission of Datascope Corp. Clinical Educational Services,
1986.

- Balloon deflates before end of diastole
- Aortic pressure rises before next systolic ejection
- Reduces coronary artery filling
- Deprives coronary arteries of adequate perfusion

Adjust timing; deflate later.

- Balloon does not deflate before next systole
- Left ventricle pumps against increased pressure
- Increases work of left ventricle
- Diminishes peak systolic pressure
- Impairs systolic ejection

Adjust timing; deflate earlier.

Insertion

- Prior to placement a clear ECG and arterial line trace must be displayed (the arterial line is best placed in the left radial artery); establish central pressure monitoring line
- Balloon insertion may be accomplished at bedside or in fluoroscopy lab
- Have pacemaker, defibrillator, and intubation equipment available during insertion
- Prepare for administration of broad-spectrum antibiotic as ordered by physician
- Select and set triggering and timing parameters
  - options of augmentation range from every beat (1:1) to every eighth beat (1:8), which facilitates adjustments necessary for a variety of clinical conditions and gradual weaning
- Check gas tank, pressure gauge
- Have X-ray available to ascertain position of balloon; radiopaque tip of catheter should be observed between the 2nd and 3rd ICS to preclude obstruction of the subclavian, mescenteric or renal arteries

Acute sudden back pain may indicate aortic dissection.

Central Aortic Pressure Monitoring

- Adhere to protocol for arterial pressure monitoring
  - heparin flush solution mixed per hospital policy
  - maintain patency of the central lumen
  - patent, leak free luer lock junctions
  - if pressure wave dampens, aspirate 3 cc of blood from central aortic pressure line; if resistance to aspiration is noted, lumen should be considered occluded and use discontinued; a sterile male luer lock cap should be placed on the port
  - maintain a central aortic pressure line according to accepted protocol for arterial line management

Bedside Management

- Patient should be on bedrest
- Elevate head of bed no more than 30°
- Minimize knee and hip flexion to prevent kinking or fracture of the balloon catheter

- Assess peripheral pulses hourly, using doppler as necessary
  - compare color, temperature, and sensitivity of catheterized and noninvolved extremities
  - monitor temperature, color, and pulses of arms, particularly on involved side (rule out balloon occlusion of left subclavian artery)
- Monitor neurological status (rule out embolus or left carotid occlusion by balloon)
- Monitor renal function (rule out occlusion of renal artery)
- Observe hemodynamic monitoring parameters
  - evaluate timing and effectiveness of counterpulsation
- Monitor lab studies, including CBC, coagulation profile, electrolytes, CXR, and ECG
- Observe for signs of bleeding or infection at insertion site
- Utilize heparin therapy (in some institutions low molecular weight dextran is used in place of heparinization)
- Observe for console failure
  - in the event of console malfunction the balloon should be manually inflated/deflated every 10 min to prevent clot formation on the balloon
- Observe for balloon rupture/gas leak
  - safety chamber for inflation failure
  - for augmentation loss (dampened waveform)
- Assess augmentation loss
  - patient status (variations in HR, B/P)
  - available gas (helium or CO_2) volume
  - timing
- Maintain strict aseptic technique and change occlusive dressing every 24 hr
- Catheter removal
  - turn console off and manually aspirate balloon to deflate it
  - after removal, assess insertion site for bleeding; evaluate peripheral pulses; maintain HOB elevation at <45°
  - bedrest recommended for 48 hr after removal of balloon

Weaning
- Reduce patient/balloon ratio from 1:1 to 1:8 over a period of time depending on patient tolerance
- Evidence of intolerance: increasing pulmonary capillary wedge pressure, decreasing mean arterial pressure, decreasing cardiac output, reduction in urinary output, dysrhythmias, or chest pain

Complications
- Nonfunctional balloon
- Balloon leak
- Excessive bleeding at insertion site
- Ischemia of affected extremity
- Infection
- Aortic dissection
- Obstruction of subclavian, renal, or mesenteric arteries
- Thrombus formation
- Thrombocytopenia

AUTOMATIC IMPLANTABLE CARDIOVERTER DEFIBRILLATOR (AICD)

Ventak® PRx® II (Model 1715) and Ventak® PRx® III (Model 1720 and 1725)

Function
- Monitor and regulate heart rate
- Sense cardiac rate
- Delivery of pacing pulses
- Delivery of defibrillating shocks

Indications
- Treatment of ventricular fibrillation and/or tachydysrhythmias capable of producing sudden cardiac death
  - survival from at least one episode of cardiac arrest as a result of hemodynamically unstable ventricular tachydysrhythmia—**NOT ASSOCIATED WITH ACUTE MYOCARDIAL INFARCTION**
  - spontaneously recurring, poorly tolerated, sustained ventricular tachycardia (VT) and/or ventricular fibrillation (VF)
  - VT or VF inducible in spite of drug therapy

Contraindications
- Ventricular tachydysrhythmias that may have a reversible cause
  - Digitalis toxicity
  - electrolyte imbalance
  - hypoxia
  - sepsis
- Ventricular tachydysrhythmias with a transient cause
  - acute myocardial infarction (AMI)
  - electrocution
  - drowning
- Patients who have, or require, a unipolar pacemaker

Patients whose ventricular dysrhythmia requires frequent shocks, the pulse generator batteries can deplete soon after implantation

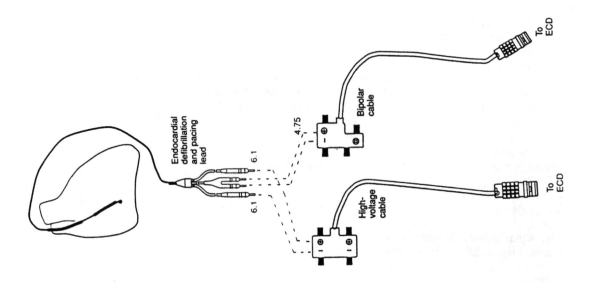

a

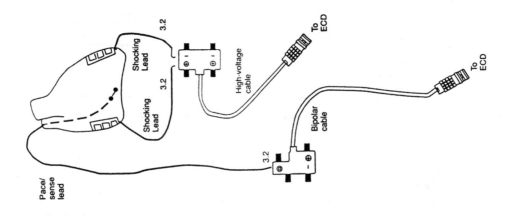

b

Figure 1.65   Lead to ECD Connections for Lead Evaluation
(a) Lead-only configuration of an ENDOTAK endocardial cardioversion/defibrillation and pacing lead;
(b) An inline endocardial pace/sense lead and two patch leads

Ventak® PRx II/PRx III Life Expectancy Estimation (Implant to ERI)[1]

Pace/Sense %	34-J Shock Frequency	Life Expectancy[2]	
		Stored EGM OFF	**Stored EGM ON**
Pacing off	Quarterly 34-J shocks	4.7 years	4.1 years
15% pacing	Monthly 34-J shocks	3.8 years	3.4 years
100% pacing	Monthly 34-J shocks	3.1 years	2.8 years

[1]Factory nominal setting: 50 ppm pacing rate, 4.0 V pacing pulse amplitude, 0.5 ms pacing pulse width, 500 Ω pacing impedance.

[2]EGM storage feature is nominally ON.

The longevity of the pulse generator decreases with an increase in the pacing rate, pacing amplitude, pacing pulse width, percentage of bradycardia paced to sensed events, or charging frequency, or with a decrease in pacing impedance. A 34-J shock is equal to approximately seven days of monitoring.

EGM = electrogram; ERI = elective replacement indicator

Reprinted with permission of Cardiac Pacemakers, Inc. (Guidant Corporation, 4100 Hamline Ave., North, St. Paul, MN 55112), from *Physician's System Manual,* 1995.

Components
- Pulse generator
- Programmer/recorder/monitor (PRM)
- CPI Model 2872 software application
- Accessory telemetry wand

Warnings
- External defibrillation may damage the AICD pulse generator
  - place defibrillation paddles as far from pulse generator as possible
  - minimize current flowing through pulse generator and leads by positioning defibrillator paddles perpendicular to the implanted pulse generator/lead system

– use lowest energy output as is clinically feasible
– confirm pulse generator function immediately following defibrillation episode
- Internal defibrillation may damage pulse generator and cause shunting of energy
    – disconnect pulse generator from leads prior to defibrillation
    – changes in patient condition, drug regimen, and other factors may change the defibrillation threshold
- **Keep patients with implanted pulse generators away from MRI devices**
    – alternating magnetic field from MRI procedures may cause a pulse generator to charge and deliver a high-voltage shock to patient, inhibit bradycardia pacing, disable antitachycardia therapy, change programmed parameters
- Medical personnel skilled in CPR and external defibrillation techniques should be present when noninvasive testing of pulse generator takes place

Never incinerate a pulse generator; it contains sealed chemical power cells and capacitors. In the event of patient death, regardless of cause, return the implanted pulse generator and leads to the manufacturer.

- **Environmental interference**
    – electrosurgical equipment (deactivate pulse generator prior to procedure)
    – ionizing radiation
    – lithotropsy
    – electric power sources
    – arc welding equipment
    – electrical smelting furnace
    – large RF transmitters, such as radar
    – therapeutic diathermy equipment
    – electronic surveillance device (anti-theft device)
    – cellular phone (effect of cellular phone on pulse generators is temporary, keep phone at least six inches from AICD)
    – leaning over the alternator of a running car

    – strong magnetic field (>0.1 tesla)
       * industrial transformers or motors
       * MRI devices
       * large stereo speakers
       * telephone receivers (held within 0.5 in or 1.27 cm of the pulse generator)
       * radio transmitter used to control toy cars or airplanes
       * magnetic wands used in airport security or in the game "bingo"

- **Adverse physical effects of implantation**
  - acceleration of dysrhythmia
  - air embolism
  - bleeding
  - nerve damage
  - tissue erosion
  - excessive scarring
  - extrusion
  - fluid accumulation
  - hematomas/cysts
  - inappropriate shocks
  - infection
  - keloid formation
  - lead abrasion, fracture, migration, dislodgment
  - myocardial damage
  - pneumothorax
  - pulse generator malfunction
  - thromboemboli
  - venous occlusion, perforation
  - cardiac perforation
  - shunting current with defibrillation

Whenever a warbling tone is heard coming from the device, patient is advised to have pulse generator checked.

VENTRICULAR ASSIST DEVICE (VAD)

The VAD is an extracorporeal blood pump that diverts circulating blood around the failing ventricle, allowing the ventricle to rest and regulating intracardiac pressures.

Types
- Left sided (LVAD)
  - cannula in left atrium and aorta
  - provides left ventricular support
- Right sided (RVAD)
  - cannula in right atrium and pulmonary artery
  - provides right ventricular support
- Biventricular assist device (BVAD)
  - cannula in right atrium, pulmonary artery, left atrium, and aorta
  - provides right *and* left ventricular support

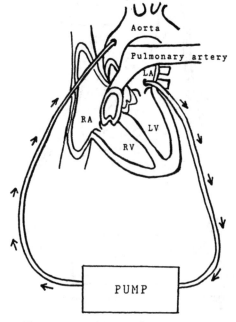

Figure 1.66 Left Ventricular Assist Device

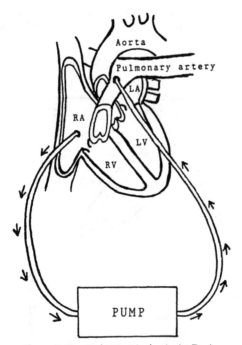

Figure 1.67   Right Ventricular Assist Device

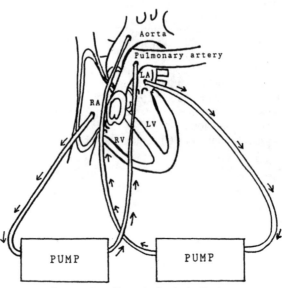

Figure 1.68   Biventricular Assist Device

Indications
- Patients awaiting cardiac transplantation
- Patients in cardiogenic shock
- Patients who have had cardiac surgery but cannot be weaned from cardiopulmonary bypass

Contraindications
- Chronic renal failure
- Symptomatic cerebral vascular disease
- Blood dyscrasia

Complications
- Thrombus formation
- Emboli
- Sepsis
- Increased metabolic demand
- Renal failure
- Fluid shift
- Neurological impairment
- Pulmonary complications (atelectasis, pneumonia)
- CHF/pulmonary edema
- Muscle atrophy, contractures, skin breakdown

Nursing/Medical Implications
- Clinical parameters that can be manipulated:
  - cardiac output (3–6 L/min)
  - heart rate (60–120 BPM)
  - systolic duration (35–45%)
  - vacuum (15–20 cm H_2O)
  - drive pressure (210–240 mm Hg)

- Effectiveness of VAD reflected in
  - B/P
  - peripheral perfusion
  - hemodynamic measurements
  - level of consciousness
  - urinary output
- Other therapies that may be used in conjunction with the VAD:
  - pharmacologic agents
  - fluid and electrolyte balance
  - IABP
- A perfusionist expert in the mechanics of extracorporeal circulation should be readily available to manage the device; the perfusionist is responsible for any adjustments
- About 30% of patients with LVAD develop right ventricular failure and require additional support (inotropic drugs or BVAD)
- Patient is usually sedated and immobilized; requires mechanical ventilation

Cardiac compressions are contraindicated, as they may dislodge the cannulae. If indicated, internal cardiac massage may be performed.

NORMAL RANGES AND VARIATIONS IN THE ADULT TWELVE-LEAD ELECTROCARDIOGRAM

A true understanding of the normal range and variation of the ECG depends on a basic understanding of both normal and abnormal cardiac electrophysiology. Many of the configurations tabulated here may represent cardiac abnormalities when interpreted in the context of the entire tracing and in light of the individual's clinical history and physical examination. Therefore the information contained in the following table is intended for use only as a rough preliminary guide to the interpretation of ambiguous and borderline tracings.

Lead	P	Q	R	S	ST	T
I	Upright.	Small (less than 0.04 s and less than 25% of R).	Dominant. Largest deflection of the QRS complex.	Less than R, or none.	Usually isoelectric; may vary from +1 to –0.5 mm.	Upright.
II	Upright.	Small or none.	Dominant.	Less than R, or none.	Usually isoelectric; may vary from +1 to –0.5 mm.	Upright.
III	Upright, flat, diphasic, or inverted, depending on frontal plane axis.	Small or none, depending on frontal plane axis; or large (0.04–0.05 s or greater than 25% of R).	None to dominant, depending on frontal plane axis.	None to dominant, depending on frontal plane axis.	Usually isoelectric; may vary from +1 to –0.5 mm.	Upright, flat, diphasic, or inverted, depending on frontal plane axis.
aVR	Inverted.	Small, none, or large.	Small or none, depending on frontal plane axis.	Dominant (may be QS).	Usually isoelectric; may vary from +1 to –0.5 mm.	Inverted.

Lead	P	Q	R	S	ST	T
aVL	Upright, flat, diphasic, or inverted, depending on frontal plane axis.	Small, none, or large, depending on frontal plane axis.	Small, none, or dominant, depending on frontal plane axis.	None to dominant, depending on frontal plane axis.	Usually isoelectric; may vary from +1 to −0.5 mm.	Upright, flat, diphasic, or inverted, depending on frontal plane axis.
aVF	Upright.	Small or none.	Small, none, or dominant, depending on frontal plane axis.	None to dominant; depending on frontal plane axis.	Usually isoelectric; may vary from +1 to −0.5 mm.	Upright, flat, diphasic, or inverted, depending on frontal plane axis.
V_1	Inverted, flat, upright, or diphasic.	None (may be QS).	Less than S, or none (QS); small r′ may be present.	Dominant (may be QS).	0 to +3 mm.	Upright, flat, diphasic, or inverted.
V_2	Upright; less commonly diphasic or inverted.	None (may be QS).	Less than S, or none (QS); small r′ may be present.	Dominant (may be QS).	0 to +3 mm.	Upright; less commonly flat; diphasic, or inverted.
V_3	Upright.	Small or none.	R less than, greater than, or equal to S.	S greater than, less than, or equal to R.	0 to +3 mm.	Upright.
V_4	Upright.	Small or none.	R greater than S.	S less than R.	Usually isoelectric; may vary from +1 to −0.5 mm.	Upright.
V_5	Upright.	Small.	Dominant (less than 26 mm).	S less than SV_4		Upright.
V_6	Upright.	Small.	Dominant (less than 26 mm).	S less than SV_5.		Upright.

Reprinted with permission from Goldschlager N, Goldman MJ: Principles of Clinical Electrocardiography, 13th ed., Norwalk, CT: Appleton & Lange, 1989.

MYOCARDIAL INFARCTION

LOCATION/EKG CHANGES

Location	Involved Vessel	Q Wave	R Wave	ST	T Wave
Anterior	LCA	Normal septal Q in I and V_6 Abnormal in V_3 and V_4	Initial in V_4R, V_3R, V_1 $\downarrow$ in amplitude of the R wave in left precordial leads	Elevation in V_1 (may extend to V_5 or V_6)	Inversion in V_1–V_4 (may extend to V_5 or V_6)
Anterolateral	LAD, circumflex	I, aVL, V_3–V_6	Loss of R in V_3–V_6	Elevation in V_4–V_6, aVL, I Downward in III	Inversion in V_4–V_6, aVL, I Upward in III
Lateral	Circumflex, branch of LAD	I, aVL, V_4–V_6		Elevation in I, aVL, V_4–V_6	Inverted in I, aVL, V_4–V_6
Anteroseptal	LAD	V_1–V_4	Loss of R wave in V_2, V_3 Present in V_4–V_6	Elevation in V_4R to V_3 or V_4	Inversion in V_4R to V_3 or V_4
Inferior	RCA	II, III, aVF		Elevation in II, III, aVF	Inversion in II, III, aVF
Posterior	RCA, LCA, circumflex	II, III, aVF	Prominent in V_1 or V_2	Elevation in I, III, aVF	Symmetric deeply inverted in I, III, aVF Usually upright in V_1
Apical	RCA, LCA	II, III, aVF; in one or more of leads V_1–V_4	Loss of normal R wave in I, V_3, V_4	Elevated in I Inverted in III	Inverted in I Elevated in III
Right ventricular (commonly observed in conjunction with inferior or posterior infarcts)	Main RCA	Right pre-cordial leads		Elevated in V_1–V_3 Elevated in right chest leads V_3R–V_6R	

Note: RCA = right coronary artery; LAD = left anterior descending; LCA = left coronary artery.

Subendocardial (nontransmural) MI diagnosis is difficult and is based on typical ischemic chest pain lasting >15 min, ST = segment depression and/or T-wave inversion >48 hr, elevated cardiac enzymes, and absence of Q waves. Transmural MI involves the entire thickness of the myocardium.

INTERVENTION IN PATIENTS WITH HEMODYNAMIC IMBALANCE: CONGESTIVE HEART FAILURE OR SHOCK

Management Goal	Intervention

1. Preload
    To decrease preload (with pulmonary or systemic congestion)
	Decrease venous return
	    High Fowler's position with legs dangling
	    Morphine sulfate
	    Diuretics (Lasix/Bumex)
	    Nitroglycerin, isosorbide (Isordil)
	      (decreases afterload also)
	    PEEP
	    Fluid restriction, decrease IV fluids

To increase preload (with decreased cardiac output and wedge)	*Increase volume*
	    Crystalloids
	    Dextran

2. To decrease afterload	Nitroprusside (Nipride) Hydralazine (Apresoline) Captopril (Capoten) IABP
3. To increase contractility	Dopamine Dobutamine Amrinone Digitalis

4. To increase O_2 supply and decrease O_2 demand	Correction of arrhythmias
	Repair of mechanical defects
	Oxygen
	Psychological support
	Rest
	Morphine sulfate
	IABP
	Ventricular assist devices
	Coronary bypass
	Decrease of preload/afterload
5. To support tissue metabolism	Hyperalimentation
	Steroids

Reprinted with permission from Crawford MV, Spence MI. *Commonsense Approach to Coronary Care,* 6th ed. St. Louis: Mosby-Year Book, Inc., 1995.

DIFFERENTIATION OF VENTRICULAR TACHYCARDIA (VT) AND SUPRAVENTRICULAR TACHYCARDIA (SVT)†

ECG	SVT	VT
• QRS morphology	• RBBB in V_1 and V_6 leads	• LBBB most common
• QRS width	• <0.14 sec	• >0.14 sec
• Axis deviation	• Left axis deviation uncommon	• Occasional left axis deviation
• AV dissociation	• Infrequent	• Frequent
• Fusion beats	• Rare	• Occasional
• Capture beats	• None	• Occasional
• Concordancy (– or + in V leads)	• Not usually present	• Strong indicator
• Preceded by	• PAC	• PVC
• Physical findings		
– Cannon waves	• Rare	• Common
– Vagal maneuver response	• Rate may slow	• No response
• Therapy		
– Lidocaine	• No response	• Response likely
– Verapamil	• Slows rate	• May get worse

---

†If definitive diagnosis does not rule out ventricular tachycardia, verapamil should be avoided; procainamide is the first choice drug.

chapter 2

RESPIRATORY EVALUATION AND MANAGEMENT

ARTIFICIAL AIRWAY DEVICES

OROPHARYNGEAL

Indications

- Airway obstruction with nasal obstruction
- High probability of epistaxis (fracture, deviated septum, etc.)
- Unconscious patient with adequate respiratory effort
- Maintenance of airway prior to intubation

Advantages/Disadvantages

- Advantages
  - short-term intubation
  - simplest airway adjunct
- Disadvantages
  - cannot be used if patient is conscious
  - may cause gagging
  - secretions may be aspirated; suctioning should be available

Nursing/Medical Implications

- Must be properly placed; improperly placed may occlude airway
- Cannot be used with lower facial trauma or oral surgery
- Respiratory status must be closely monitored

NASOPHARYNGEAL (NASAL TRUMPET)

Indications

- Airway obstruction with trauma to jaw or lower face
- Oral surgery
- Maintenance of airway after anesthesia

Advantages/Disadvantages

- Advantages
  - can be used in alert, conscious patient
- Disadvantages
  - secretions may be aspirated; suctioning should be available
  - may become clogged
  - may not be used if nares is obstructed
  - may not be used if patient prone to nose bleeds

Nursing/Medical Implications

- Airway should be changed every 6–8 hr to prevent ulceration of mucous membranes
- Respiratory status must be closely monitored

ORAL ENDOTRACHEAL INTUBATION
Indications
- Short-term airway management requiring mechanical ventilation
  - CPR
  - respiratory insufficiency/failure
  - removal of airway secretions
- Need to deliver an FIO_2 >60%

Advantages/Disadvantages
- Advantages
  - prevents damage to nasal passage
  - shorter, larger diameter tube used; lessens airway resistance and mucous plugging
  - facilitates tracheobronchial suctioning
  - best device for emergency
- Disadvantages
  - only trained persons may insert
  - poorly tolerated, requires sedation
  - may not be used after oral or dental surgery, major facial trauma
  - may cause damage to vocal cords
  - subglottic stenosis
  - requires alternate means of communication

Nursing/Medical Implications
- Suction equipment must be readily available
- Tube placement must be verified by chest X-ray
- Tube may slip into bronchus, cutting off air to opposite lung
- Tube requires careful stabilization
- May require oral airway to prevent patient biting tube
- Patient will try to remove tube by whatever method; may require protective restraint

NASAL ENDOTRACHEAL INTUBATION

Indications

- Long-term airway management (>48 hr)
  - respiratory insufficiency/failure
  - removal of airway secretions
  - lower facial trauma

Advantages/Disadvantages

- Advantages
  - better tolerated by patients; less sedation required
  - patient able to swallow
  - tube easily stabilized
  - patient less apt to extubate self
- Disadvantages
  - only trained persons may insert
  - smaller diameter, longer tube may make bronchoscopy more difficult
  - smaller tube more likely to become clogged
  - suctioning may be more difficult
  - may not be used with nasal, sinus fractures or cerebrospinal fluid leak
  - may cause damage to vocal cords, necrosis of the nasal septum
  - subglottic stenosis
  - requires alternative method of communication

Nursing/Medical Implications

- Tube may slip into bronchus, cutting off air supply to opposite lung
- Suction equipment must be readily available
- Suctioning not as effective as with oral intubation
- Tube placement must be verified by chest X-ray

TRACHEOSTOMY

Indications

- Long-term intubation
- When endotracheal intubation impossible
- Complete upper airway obstruction

Advantages/Disadvantages

- Advantages
  - short, wide tube produces less resistance, increased patient comfort
  - better tolerated
  - mucous plugging less likely
  - suctioning easier, more effective
  - easy stabilization of cannula
  - precludes damage to oral, nasal, pharyngeal, laryngeal structures
- Disadvantages
  - surgical procedure requiring anesthesia
  - increased danger of infection
  - contraindicated in patients with fresh sternotomy

Nursing/Medical Implications

- If extubation occurs during first 24 hr, reinsertion of tube may be difficult
- If extubation occurs after 48 hr, replacement may be accomplished without difficulty
- Weaning from ventilator less stressful than with oro/nasotracheal intubation
- Suction equipment must be readily available

ESOPHAGEAL OBTURATOR AIRWAY (EOA)

Indications

- Emergency situations requiring airway establishment
- Short-term airway management

Advantages/Disadvantages

- Advantages
  - may be inserted by persons untrained in endotracheal intubation; little technical skill required
  - visualization not required for insertion
  - prevents aspiration of vomitus

Nursing/Medical Implications

- EOA should be used only as an interim method of airway management
- Endotracheal intubation must be accomplished as quickly as possible

Indications

Advantages/Disadvantages

  – may be used on persons with
    cervical spine injury; placed with
    head in a neutral position
  – facilitates endotracheal
    intubation
• Disadvantages
  – cannot be used if patient
    conscious or semiconscious
  – contraindicated in patients who
    have ingested caustic substances
    or who have esophageal disease
    or foreign body in trachea

Nursing/Medical Implications

• Suctioning equipment must be
  readily available when EOA is
  removed; vomiting is a frequent
  occurrence
• May be accidentally positioned in
  trachea

If so, remove it immediately.

CRICOTHYROTOMY
Indications

• Immediate (urgent) airway access
  when translaryngeal approach is
  not feasible
  – facial trauma
  – inhalation burns
  – glottic edema
  – fractured larynx
  – foreign body at glottis

Advantages/Disadvantages

• Advantages
  – rapid entry into an obstructed
    airway
  – cuffed tube may be inserted
  – buys time for transtracheal
    intubation
• Disadvantages
  – possibility of hemorrhage,
    laceration of the esophagus,
    tracheal stenosis
  – false passage of tube
  – subcutaneous/mediastinal
    emphysema may result

Nursing/Medical Implications

• May be accomplished by incision
  or in some cases with a 12–14-
  gauge, 8.5-cm needle

**An *absolute* emergency procedure
that should *never* be attempted if
a more conservative procedure is
possible (i.e., transtracheal
intubation, naso/oropharyngeal
airway, EOA)**

OXYHEMOGLOBIN DISSOCIATION CURVE

Oxygen bound to hemoglobin = Hgb concentration × 1.34 × % O_2 saturation (1.34 is the greatest amount of O_2 in mL that can be bound to 1 g of hemoglobin)

$$O_2 \text{ content (mL/100 mL blood)} = \frac{(Hg)\ (1.34)(Hb\ O_2\ Sat)}{100} + (PaO_2)(0.003)$$

PaO_2 = partial pressure of arterial oxygen

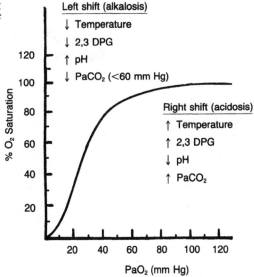

Left shift (alkalosis)
↓ Temperature
↓ 2,3 DPG
↑ pH
↓ $PaCO_2$ (<60 mm Hg)

Right shift (acidosis)
↑ Temperature
↑ 2,3 DPG
↓ pH
↑ $PaCO_2$

Figure 2.1 Oxyhemoglobin Dissociation Curve

ARTERIAL/ALVEOLAR (a/A) RATIO

To calculate alveolar O_2 tension:

$$\textbf{Step 1} \quad P_AO_2 = FIO_2 \times (Pb - PH_2O) - \frac{PaCO_2}{RQ}$$

$$\textbf{Step 2} \quad PaO_2 \div P_AO_2$$

The difference between calculated P_AO_2 and measured PaO_2 is normally less than 10–15 mm Hg.

- P_AO_2 = partial pressure of alveolar oxygen
- PaO_2 = partial pressure of arterial oxygen
- FIO_2 = fraction of inspired oxygen
- Pb = barometric pressure (assumed to be 760 mm Hg at sea level)
- PH_2O = water pressure in the lungs (assumed to be 47 mm Hg)
- $PaCO_2$ = partial pressure of carbon dioxide in arterial blood
- RQ = respiratory quotient (assumed to be 0.8)

SUPPLEMENTAL OXYGEN DEVICES

NASAL CANNULA[†]

Flow Rate L/min	% of O$_2$ Delivered	Advantages	Disadvantages
1	22–24	• Convenient, comfortable	• Can be used only in patients with adequate breathing function
2	26–28	• Low cost	• Nasal passages must be patent
3	28–30	• Allows patient mobility	• Dries mucous membranes
4	32–36	• Allows patient to eat, drink, talk	• May cause pressure areas over ears, under nose
5	36–40	• Practical for long-term therapy	• Should not exceed 6 L/min
6	40–44	• No rebreathing of expired air	
		• Concentration of O$_2$ delivered not affected by mouth breathing	

NASAL CATHETER[†]

Flow Rate L/min	% of O$_2$ Delivered	Advantages	Disadvantages
1	22–24	• Allows freedom of movement	• Less comfortable than nasal cannula
2	26–28	• Allows patient to eat, drink, talk	• May cause abdominal distention
3	28–30	• Inexpensive, disposable	• Dries mucous membranes
4	32–36		• May become clogged with secretions
5	36–40		• Should be changed every 6–8 hours, alternating nares
6	40–44		• Good for short-term therapy
			• Should not exceed 6 L/min

[†]Low-flow system.

OXYMIZER—OXYGEN-CONSERVING DEVICE[†]

Flow Rate L/min	% of O_2 Delivered
.5	20.4
1.0	25.4
1.5	29.6
2.0	34.6
2.5	38.8
3.0	43.0
3.5	47.2
4.0	51.3
4.5	55.5
5.0	59.5
5.5	63.6
6.0	68.0
6.5	72.1
7.0	76.3
7.5	80.3

Advantages

- Reduced oxygen cost
- Enhances patient mobility
- Reduces nasal irritation, dryness
- Eliminates need for humidification
- Allows use of low-volume oxygen concentrators by high-flow patients
- Adequately saturates higher-flow patient without oxygen mask

Disadvantages

- Patient must have adequate breathing function
- Nasal passages must be patent
- Should be replaced about every 3 weeks or more frequently as needed for for sanitation, depending on the conditions of use

[†]Reprinted with permission of Chad Therapeutics, Inc. (9445 De Soto Ave., Chatsworth, CA 91311), 1995.

SIMPLE FACE MASK[†]

Flow Rate L/min	% of O_2 Delivered
5	40
6	45–50
8	55–60

Advantages
- Higher O_2 concentration delivered than by nasal cannula
- Doesn't dry mucous membranes

Disadvantages
- Patient must have spontaneous breathing
- Confining
- Poorly tolerated by dyspneic patient
- May irritate skin
- Interferes with eating and drinking
- May cause pressure areas on bony facial parts
- Requires flow rate ≥5 L/min
- Impractical for long-term therapy

VENTURI MASK[‡]

Flow Rate L/min	% of O_2 Delivered
Blue: 4	24
Yellow: 4–6	28
White: 6–8	31
Green: 8–10	35
Pink: 8–12	40
Orange: 12	50

Advantages
- Delivers an exact O_2 concentration
- The FIO_2 dial can be changed to deliver a calculated O_2 concentration
- Can be used to deliver humidity or aerosol therapy

Disadvantages
- Patient must be breathing spontaneously
- May irritate skin
- Interferes with eating, drinking
- Tight seal should be maintained around nose and mouth
- Confining
- FIO_2 concentration may be lowered if air intake ports are occluded

---

[†]Low-flow system.

[‡]High-flow system.

NONREBREATHER[†]

Flow Rate L/min	% of O$_2$ Delivered
6	55–60
8	60–80
10	80–90
12–15	90

Advantages

- Delivers highest possible O$_2$ concentration
- Doesn't dry mucous membranes
- May be converted to partial rebreather if needed
- Has one-way expiratory valve that prevents rebreathing expired gases

Disadvantages

- Patient must have spontaneous respirations
- Uncomfortable, confining
- Tight seal necessary
- May irritate skin
- Impractical for long-term therapy
- Bag must not be twisted or totally deflated
- Rubber diaphragms on mask must remain intact
- May cause O$_2$ toxicity; monitor ABGs
- Interferes with eating, drinking, talking

[†]Low-flow system.
[‡]High-flow system.

PARTIAL REBREATHER[†]

Flow Rate L/min	% of O_2 Delivered
6	35
8	40–50
10–15	60

Advantages
- Increased fraction of inspired O_2 (FIO$_2$)
- Delivers high O_2 concentrations
- Doesn't dry mucous membranes
- May be converted to a nonbreather if needed
- Safety valve allows inhalation of room air if O_2 source fails

Disadvantages
- Patient must have spontaneous respirations
- Hot/confining
- May irritate skin
- Tight seal necessary
- Interferes with eating, drinking, talking
- Not practical for long-term therapy
- Bag must not be twisted or totally deflated

FACE TENT[§]

Flow Rate L/min	% of O_2 Delivered
15	40–100

Advantages
- Can be used in place of a face mask if patient cannot tolerate having nose covered (fracture, nasal surgery, anxiety)
- Doesn't dry mucous membranes
- Delivers precise O_2 concentration when attached to venturi system

Disadvantages
- Patient must have spontaneous respirations
- Interferes with eating, drinking
- Hot but less confining than face mask
- May irritate skin
- Impractical for long-term therapy

[†]Low-flow system.

[§]High- or low-flow system. Functions as a high-flow system when attached to a venturi nebulizer.

T-TUBE[§§]

Flow Rate L/min	% of O_2 Delivered
15	40–100

Advantages
- Offers high humidity
- Can be used on tracheostomy or endotracheal tube
- Allows greater patient mobility during weaning
- Functions as high-flow system when attached to venturi components

Disadvantages
- Condensation builds up in system
- May cause O_2 toxicity

TRACH COLLAR/MASK[†]

Flow Rate L/min	% of O_2 Delivered
15	40–100

Advantages
- Provides high humidity
- Swivel adapter allows mobility; may be attached from either side
- May be suctioned from frontal port (exhalation port)

Do not cover this port.

Disadvantages
- Condensation builds up in system and may drain into tracheostomy
- Secretions may collect in collar; set up for infection of stoma
- Intake of room air through frontal port lowers O_2 concentration

---

[§§]High- or low-flow system.
[†]Low-flow system.

PULSE OXIMETRY

Arterial pulse oximetry continuously monitors the arterial oxygen saturation of blood, without trauma or discomfort.

Indications
- Patients at risk for poor perfusion
  - COPD
  - CHF
  - ARDS
  - head trauma
  - stroke
  - open-heart surgery
- Rapid desaturation states
  - fever
  - dyspnea
  - anxiety
  - agitation
  - weaning from ventilator
  - suctioning

Disadvantages
- Physiological/environmental variables that produce derangement in oximetry readings
  - dye used in cardiac output studies
  - dyshemoglobin (carboxyhemoglobin, methemoglobin, etc.)
  - elevated bilirubin concentrations of >20%
  - poor tissue perfusion
- Measures only O_2 concentrations

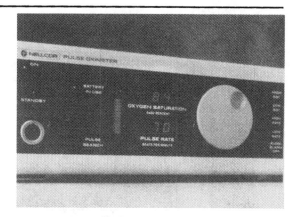

Figure 2.2 Pulse Oximeter

Reprinted with permission of Nellcor Incorporated (4280 Hacienda Drive, Pleasanton, CA 94588), 1995.

CAPNOGRAPHY

Capnography is the measurement of carbon dioxide concentration in expired respiratory gas. Waveforms are produced by changing levels of carbon dioxide. These changes afford the clinician a viable means of assessing airway and cardiopulmonary/metabolic systems. Alterations in patient condition may be recognized before clinical signs or symptoms are apparent.

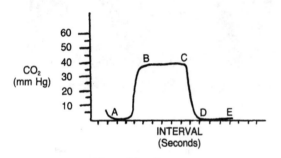

Figure 2.3 Capnogram

A = beginning expiration (baseline).

B = plateau onset.

C = end of plateau. End of expiratory phase/beginning of inspiratory phase; best approximation of alveolar CO_2.

BC = alveolar CO_2 outflow.

CD = during inspiration CO_2 decreases.

DE = remainder of inspiration.

End tidal value is approximately 38 mm Hg.

Indications
- Assessment of clinical condition to determine need for mechanical ventilation
- Validation of endotracheal tube placement
- Adjustment of ventilator setting
- Reduces need for ABGs
- Identifies leaks in respiratory circuit, kinked tubing, disconnections
- Facilitates diagnosis of
  - pulmonary embolus
  - pneumothorax
  - hemorrhage
  - shock
- Assessment of ventilatory status in
  - asthma, COPD, atelectasis
  - drug overdose
  - cardiopulmonary resuscitation

Type	Advantages	Disadvantages
Mainstream • Special airway adapter with measurement sensor	• Results obtained quickly • Automatically calibrated, using a cell that contains a mixture of CO_2 and nitrogen	• Can be used only on an intubated patient • Added dead space • Expensive measurement sensor required • Measurement sensor exposed to environmental damage
Sidestream • Gas routed through a capillary to capnometer	• May be used on a nonintubated patient • Carbon dioxide measurement chamber protected inside unit • Gas sampled close to patient's mouth	• Measurement delayed because of length of sample tubing • Sample tube may become clogged • Analysis takes longer

ARTERIAL BLOOD GASES

NORMAL VALUE RANGES

pH = 7.35–7.45 HCO_2 = 22–26 mEq/L
PCO_2 = 35–45 mm Hg   Base Excess (BE) = –2 to + 2
PO_2 = 80–90 mm Hg O_2 Saturation = 95–99%

INTERPRETATION OF VALUES

Status	pH	PCO_2	HCO_3	BE
Respiratory Acidosis				
Uncompensated	↓ 7.35	↑ 45	Normal	Normal
Partially compensated	↓ 7.35	↑ 45	↑ 27	↑ + 2
Compensated	7.35–7.45	↑ 45	↑ 27	↑ + 2
Respiratory Alkalosis				
Uncompensated	↑ 7.45	↓ 35	Normal	Normal
Partially compensated	↑ 7.45	↓ 35	↓ 22	↓ – 2
Compensated	7.40–7.45	↓ 35	↓ 22	↓ – 2
Metabolic Acidosis				
Uncompensated	↓ 7.35	Normal	↓ 22	↓ – 2
Partially compensated	↓ 7.35	↓ 35	↓ 22	↓ – 2
Compensated	7.35–7.40	↓35	↓ 22	↓ – 2
Metabolic Alkalosis				
Uncompensated	↑ 7.45	Normal	↑ 27	↑ + 2
Partially compensated	↑ 7.45	↑ 45	↑ 27	↑ + 2
Compensated	7.40–7.45	↑ 45	↑ 27	↑ + 2

MECHANICAL VENTILATION TYPES

	Mechanism	**Use**
Volume Cycled	• Delivers a preset volume of gas with each inspiration • Terminates inspiration after preset volume is delivered, regardless of airway pressure • Capable of developing a pressure that can maintain tidal volume when changes in resistance or compliance occur	• Most commonly used ventilator • Patients presenting problems of resistance or compliance
Time Cycled	• A given volume of gas is delivered over a predetermined (set) time interval • Inspiratory time remains constant • Volume delivered during the predetermined inspiratory time is directly related to length of inspiratory phase	• Used primarily with infants and children
Pressure Cycled	• Delivers a preset pressure to the lungs • Inspiratory flow ceases when preset pressure has been delivered • Volume of air varies with lung compliance • Depth of inspiration determined by preset pressure	• Short-term ventilator therapy (postoperative, anesthesia recovery) **This type is contraindicated for patients with lung disease and problems with compliance/ resistance.**

High-Frequency Jet Ventilator
(This type is still under clinical
   evaluation.)

Mechanism
- Delivers 40–150 breaths/min, with
  low tidal volume (up to 300 mL)
  under pressure
- Inspiration ends when preset time
  cycle elapses
- Employs fast rate/low volume

Use
- Decreases risk of barotrauma
  (pneumothorax, tracheo-
  esophageal fistulae)
- Bronchopleural fistula
- Flail chest/thoracic trauma

MODES

Control Mode Ventilation (CMV)

Mechanism
- Ventilator delivers preset tidal volume
  - rate
  - depth
- Patient has no control in ventilation cycle

Assist Control Mode (AC)
- Ventilator initiates inspiration in response to patient created negative
  pressure in circuitry

**Intermittent Mandatory
Ventilation (IMV)**
- Patient breathes spontaneously through ventilator circuitry
- At a preset interval, ventilator-assisted breath is delivered at set tidal volume
- Independent spontaneous ventilation

**Synchronized Intermittent
Mandatory Ventilation (SIMV)**
- Patient breathes spontaneously through ventilator circuitry
- Preset ventilator breath delivered with spontaneously initiated breath

**Positive End Expiratory Pressure
(PEEP)**
- Airway pressure greater than normal maintained at end of exhalation

**Continuous Positive Airway
Pressure (CPAP)**
- Application of PEEP during inspiration and expiration in spontaneously
  breathing patient

Pressure Support
- A support mode utilized for patients with intact respiratory drive
- Support mode with a constant respiratory pressure and decelerating flow

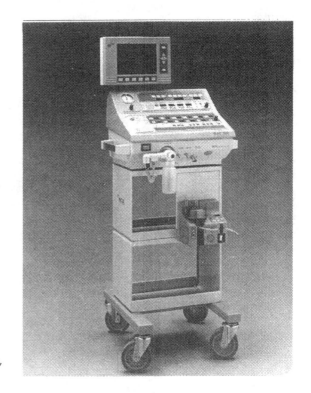

Figure 2.4A BEAR® 1000 Ventilator

Reprinted with permission from Allied Healthcare Products, Inc.—Ventilation Products Division, Riverside, CA.

BEAR® 1000 VENTILATOR SETTINGS
Monitor-Alarms

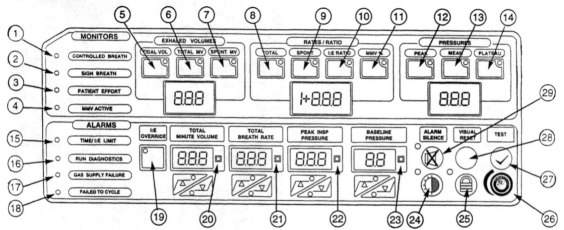

Figure 2.4B   Monitor-Alarms

Reprinted with permission from Allied Healthcare Products, Inc.—Ventilation Products Division, Riverside, CA

① **Controlled Breath**—Indicator lights whenever a Volume-Controlled, Pressure Augmented, or Pressure-Controlled breath is delivered

② **Sign Breath**—Indicator lights *only* during inspiration phase of a delivered Sigh breath

③ **Patient Effort**—Indicator lights whenever the patient exerts an effort which is equal to or greater than the clinician-selected Assist Sensitivity level

④ **MMV Active**—Indicator lights continuously during both inspiration and expiration whenever the MMV backup rate is active

⑤ **Tidal Volume**—Displays the exhaled Tidal Volume of the last breath, regardless of breath type

⑥ **Total Minute Volume**—Displays measured exhaled Minute Volume for all breaths, both demand and machine-controlled

⑦ **Spontaneous Minute Volume**—Displays measured exhaled Minute Volume for all demand breaths, including both Spontaneous and Pressure supported

⑧ **Total**—Displays the number of breaths inspired per minute, including both demand and Machine-Controlled breaths

⑨ **Spontaneous**—Displays the number of demand breaths inspired per minute; both spontaneous and Pressure-Supported breaths are included as "Demand Breaths"

⑩ **I:E Ratio**—Displays the ratio of inspiratory time to expiratory time for Volume-Controlled and Pressure-Controlled breaths *only*

⑪ **MMV%**—Displays the percentage of time during the last half hour that the MMV back-up rate has been used rather than the normal breath rate control

⑫ **Peak**—Displays the peak pressure reading during the inspiratory phase of the last positive pressure breath (e.g., Volume-Controlled, Pressure-Supported, or Pressure-Controlled, **but not spontaneous breaths**)

⑬ **Mean**—Displays the average pressure at the patient wye over the last 30-sec period

⑭ **Plateau**—Displays the inspiratory plateau pressure during the previous breath; a plateau of 0.1 sec is sufficient to create a reading

⑮ **Time/I:E Limit**—Indicator lights and alarm sounds when inspiratory time exceeds the sum of 5 sec plus the inspiratory pause time or the I:E ratio reaches the set limit; set I:E ratio is normally 1:1

(16) **Run Diagnostics**—Indicator lights **if** a major subsystem or electronic failure is detected; troubleshooting code will be displayed in Total Minute Volume LED Display by pressing the Test key

(17) **Gas Supply Failure**—Indicator lights and alarm sounds when the Gas Supply pressure drops below 27.5 PSIG

(18) **Failed to Cycle**—Indicator lights and alarm sounds if the ventilator fails to cycle due to an internal or external condition

(19) **I:E Override**—Indicator lights when key is pressed allowing override of normal 1:1 limit (Inverse ratio ventilator enabled—4:1)

(20) **Total Minute Volume**—When either of these settings is violated, an alarm sounds and the indicator flashes; low minute Volume alarm setting and MMV option can provide back-up ventilation

(21) **Total Breath Rate**—When either of these settings is violated, an alarm sounds and the indicator flashes

(22) **Peak Inspiratory Pressure**—A violation of either of these settings will cause an alarm to sound and the indicator to flash; low alarm cannot be set below 3 cm H_2O. High alarm limit violation *terminates* the breath

(23) **Baseline Pressure**—When either of these settings is violated, an alarm sounds and the indicator flashes; low alarm limit violation indicates loss of PEEP, while high alarm limit violation can indicate air trapping

(24) **Dimmer**—This key adjusts the brightness level of all front LEDs; two brightness levels are provided

(25) **Alarm Lock**—When the LED next to this key is lit, no setting changes can be made to alarm group; limits are still visible by depressing the associated key

(26) **Set Knob**—This knob is used in conjunction with high and low alarm limit keys to adjust settings; an audible tone indicates the end of the range

(27) **Test**—When depressed, it activates all audible and visual indicators for 4 sec; also used to display troubleshooting codes in Total Minute Volume display, and is used to enter operator diagnostics on power-up

(28) **Visual Reset**—Depressing this key clears all "solid" lit alarm indicators

(29) **Alarm Silence**—Cancels the audible portion of an alarm for 60 sec, except for failed-to-cycle alarm

Controls

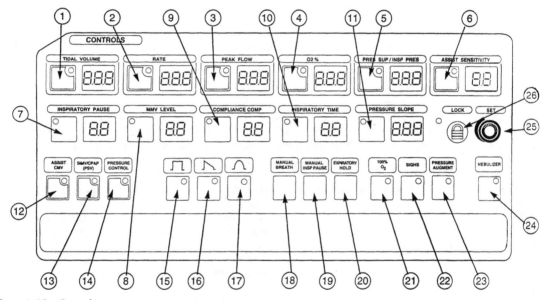

Figure 2.4C Controls

Reprinted with permission from Allied Healthcare Products, Inc.—Ventilation Products Division, Riverside, CA.

(1) **Tidal Volume (0.1 to 2.0 liters)**—Machine delivered Tidal Volume key is available in all modes except the Pressure Control mode; delivered tidal volume may exceed set tidal volume if compliance comp is in use. Tidal volume setting represents STPD (Standard Temperature 77°F, ambient pressure, DRY)

(2) **Rate (0.0, 0.5 to 120)**—Machine breath rate control is available in all modes. During CPAP, this control is set to zero

(3) **Peak Flow (10–150 LPM)**—Operates in conjunction with the waveform key to modulate the inspiratory flow pattern delivered to the patient during a volume machine breath

(4) **O₂% (21–100%)**—Determines the oxygen concentration delivered to the patient during all breath types

(5) **Pres Sup/Insp Pres (0–80 cm H₂O)**—Determines Inspiratory pressure level during a Pressure-Supported, a Pressure-Controlled, or a Pressure-Augmented breath; active as soon as the Pre Sup/Insp Pres is set above 0

(6) **Assist Sensitivity (0.2–5.0 cm H₂O)**—Determines the amount of Inspiratory effort the patient must exert to trigger a Volume-Controlled, a Pressure-Controlled, or a Pressure-Supported breath; for a Spontaneous breath to be recorded on the rate monitor, the patient must reach the assist trigger level

(7) **Inspiratory Pause (0.0–2.0 sec)**—Displays the opening of the exhalation valve after the preset tidal volume has been delivered; long pause times may lead to an I:E limit alarm

(8) **MMV Level (0–50 LPM)**—Establishes a minimum minute volume level in the SIMV and CPAP modes for backup ventilation (MMV Level ÷ Tidal Volume = Backup Rate); backup ventilation ceases when monitored exhaled minute volume exceeds MMV level by 1 LPM or 10%

(9) **Compliance Comp (0.0–7.5 ml/cm H₂O)**—Available in all modes except Pressure-Controlled; compensates for volume loss due to delivery circuit compliance; compliance compensation volume is subtracted from displayed exhaled volume

(10) **Inspiratory Time (0.1–5.0 sec)**—Active in Pressure-Controlled mode *only;* establishes the length of time during which the Inspiratory Pressure is maintained at the sum of Pres Sup/Insp Pres plus PEEP

(11) **Pressure Slope (–9 to P+9 and P–9 to P+9)**—Available in all modes; changes the speed with which the Inspiratory Pressure level is achieved, thereby influencing the degree of patient comfort (Increased ventilator/Patient synchrony)

(12) **Assist CMV**—Assist CMV LED illuminates to indicate the ventilator is operating in the assist controlled mechanical ventilation mode

⑬ **SIMV/CPAP (PSV)**—SIMV/CPAP (PSV) LED illuminates to indicate the ventilator is operating in the SIMV or CPAP mode depending on breath rate setting; additionally, Pressure-Support can be implemented in the SIMV/CPAP mode

⑭ **Pressure Control**—Pressure control LED illuminates to indicate the ventilator is operating in the Pressure-Control mode

⑮ **Square Waveform**—The square waveform causes constant flow delivery at the clinician-selected Peak Flow for the entire inspiratory phase of the breath

⑯ **Decelerating Waveform**—The Decelerating Waveform causes the flow to rapidly reach its set peak flow level, and then decrease linearly until it reaches approximately 50% of its peak

⑰ **Sine Waveform**—The Sine Waveform causes the flow to increase from zero to the peak flow setting and back to zero in a sinusoidal pattern during the inspiratory phase of a breath

⑱ **Manual Breath**—available in all modes; trigger one breath (Volume cycled or Pressure-Controlled) when pressed

⑲ **Manual Insp Pause**—Triggers a pause at end inspiration, only while control is being pressed, or 2 sec max for purposes of obtaining a plateau pressure, which is necessary for calculating compliance

⑳ **Expiratory Hold**—Only while control is being pressed, will delay breath delivery (9 sec max) for purposes of measuring intrinsic PEEP (Auto PEEP)

㉑ **100% O_2**—Press the 100% O_2 to set the blender to deliver pure oxygen to the patient until the key is pressed again or the 3-min time limit elapses

㉒ **Sighs**—Available in all modes except Pressure-Control; once activated, will deliver 1 breath every 100 breaths at 150% of set tidal volume

㉓ **Pressure Augment**—Available in all modes except Pressure-Control; effectively allows the clinician to pressure augment a volume breath, thus providing a Pressure-Supported volume-guaranteed breath

㉔ **Nebulizer**—Effectively operates during the inspiratory phase of any breath type, even spontaneously and Pressure-Supported breaths while the flow exceeds 20 LPM; automatically turns off after 30 min has elapsed

㉕ **Set Knob**—This set knob is used to adjust setting level of the upper-control group keys; an audible tone indicates the end of the range

㉖ **Control Lock**—Control lock helps avoid inadvertent changes to upper- and lower-control group settings; when LED is lit, no changes can be made to control group keys; Manual Breath and 100% O_2 can still be used

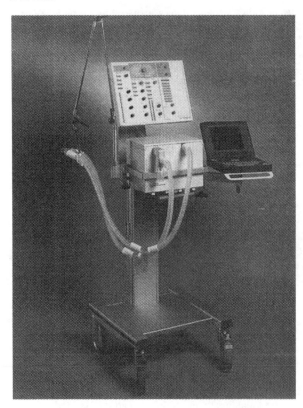

Figure 2.5A   Servo 300 Ventilator

Reprinted with permission of Siemens Medical Systems, Electromedical Group (16 Electronics Ave., Danvers, MA 01923), 1995.

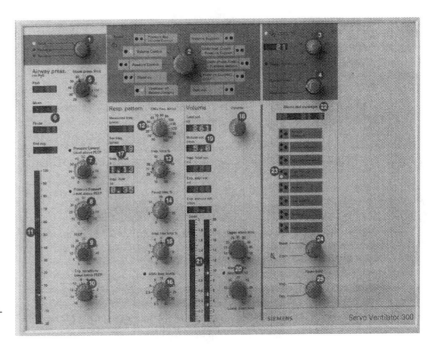

Figure 2.5B Functions of the Servo 300 Ventilator

Reprinted with permission of Siemens Medical Systems, Electromedical Group (16 Electronics Ave., Danvers, MA 01923), 1995.

FUNCTIONS OF THE SERVO 300 VENTILATOR

Patient range ① Selection of Adult, Pediatric, or Neonate

Ventilation mode ② Selection of mode:
- Battery charging, stand by
- Controlled ventilation: Pressure Control, Volume Control,
- Pressure Regulated Volume Control (new)
- Supported ventilation: Volume Support (new)
- SIMV + Pressure Support, Pressure Controlled SIMV + Pressure Support (new), Pressure Support/CPAP

O_2 concentration ③ Setting of O_2 concentration and digital display of set concentration

④ Start of oxygen breath cycle or manual start of breath

Airway pressure ⑤ Setting of Upper pressure limit

⑥ Digital display of measured values

⑦ Setting of Pressure Control level above PEEP

⑧ Setting of Pressure Support level above PEEP

⑨ Setting of PEEP level

⑩ Setting of Triggering sensitivity level below PEEP

⑪ Bar graph display of set and measured values

Respiratory pattern ⑫ Setting of CMV frequency and digital display of measured frequency

⑬ Setting of Inspiration time

⑭ Setting of Pause time

⑮ Setting of Inspiration Rise time

⑯ Setting of SIMV frequency (L/min)

⑰ Digital display of set and calculated values

Volume   (18) Setting of tidal and minute volumes

(19) Digital display of set and measured tidal and minute volumes

(20) Setting of minute volume alarm limits

(21) Bar graph display of set and measured minute volume and set minute alarm limits

Alarms and messages   (22) Message display for measured O_2 concentration or alarm messages given in full alphanumeric text

(23) Alarm table: airway pressure, O_2 concentration, expired minute volume, apnea, gas supply, battery, and technical alarms

(24) Alarm reset or alarm mute for 2 min

Pause hold   (25) Inspiration or expiration pause hold (e.g., during X-ray, auto-PEEP measurement)

Technical Specifications of Servo 300 Ventilator

General[+]

Patient unit	W 242 × D 370 × H 240 mm
Control unit	W 431 × D 150 × H 325 mm
Weight	Approx. 24 kg
Patient range	Neonate/Pediatric/Adult
Method of triggering	Flow and Pressure
Gas module flow range	0.1 ml/s–3 l/s
Settable flow range	4 ml/s–3 l/s

Gas and Power Supply

Inlet gas pressure	2–6.5 bar (29–94 PSI), air and O_2
Gas delivery system	Microprocessor-controlled valves
Power supply	100, 120, 220, and 240 V AC ± 10%
	50–60 Hz
Battery back-up time	Approx. 25 min
Recharge time	Approx. 6 h
External battery input	24 V DC
Power consumption	50 W (stand alone)

Communication/Interface

Serial port	RS-232C communication
Analog terminal	For analog outputs
Master/slave connection	For ILV (Independent Lung Ventilation) synchronization
Auxiliary equipment	For optional equipment

Modes

Controlled ventilation:

Pressure Control	Pressure-controlled ventilation
Volume Control	Volume-controlled ventilation
Pressure Reg. Volume Control	Pressure-regulated volume-controlled ventilation

[+]All dimensions in mm.

Supported ventilation:
    Volume Support   Volume-supported ventilation
    SIMV (Vol. Contr.) + Pressure   Synchronized Intermittent Mandatory Ventilation based on volume-
        Support   controlled ventilation with pressure support
    SIMV (Press. Contr.) + Pressure   Synchronized Intermittent Mandatory Ventilation based on pressure-
        Support   controlled ventilation with pressure support
    Pressure Support   Pressure-supported ventilation
    CPAP   Continuous Positive Airway Pressure ventilation
    Other settings   Ventilator off/Battery charging; Stand by

Control settings

CMV frequency	5–150 breaths/min
SIMV frequency	0.5–40 breaths/min
Inspiratory time	10–80% of breath cycle time (stepless)
Pause time	0–30% of breath cycle time (stepless)
Pressure control	0–100 cm H_2O
Pressure support	0–100 cm H_2O
PEEP	0–50 cm H_2O
Trigger sensitivity:	
Flow	3–32 ml/s (green marked area)
Pressure	–17–0 cm H_2O)
Trigger bias flow	Neonate: 8ml/s (0.5 l/min)
	Pediatric: 16 ml/s (1 l/min)
	Adult: 32 ml/s (2 l/min)
Inspiratory rise time	0–10% of breath cycle time (stepless)
Preset Tidal Volume	2–4000 ml
Preset Minute Volume	0.2–60 l/min
Oxygen breaths	100% for 20 breaths or max 1 min
Start breath	Initiation of 1 breath in all modes

Technical Specifications of Servo 300 Ventilator

Control settings (continued)

Insp. pause hold	Max 5 s
Exp. pause hold	Max 30 s
Patient range	Neonate/Pediatric/Adult
Oxygen concentration	21–100%

Alarms

Airway pressure (upper)	15–120 cm H$_2$O
High continuous pressure	Yes
O$_2$ concentration (high and low)	Set value ± 6%
Expired minute volume	
Upper alarm limit	Adult/Pediatric: 0–60 l/min
	Neonate: 0–6 l/min
Lower alarm limit	Adult/Pediatric: 0.3–40 l/min
	Neonate: 0.06–4 l/min
Apnea	10 s (Neonate)
	15 s (Pediatric)
	20 s (Adult)
Gas supply	Yes
Battery	Yes
Technical	Yes
Alarm silence	2 min
Alarm reset	Yes

Monitoring

Frequency (breath cycle time)	Set (CMV or SIMV)
Frequency	Measured
Pressure:	
Peak, Mean, Pause, End exp.	Measured
Airway pressure	Measured

Volume: Insp. Tidal Vol., Exp. Tidal Vol., Exp. Minute Vol.	Measured
Insp. Period (I:E ratio)	Set
Flow rates (l/s or l/min)	Set
O_2 concentration	Set
O_2 concentration	Measured
Supply pressure	Measured (air and O_2)
Battery voltage	Measured (internal and external)

In the Servo Ventilator 300, flow measurements and all preset and indicated volumes are referenced to standard pressure (1013 mbar, 760 mm Hg).

Servo Ventilator 300 Technical Specifications reprinted with permission of Siemens Medical Systems, Electromedical Group (16 Electronics Ave., Danvers, MA 01923), January 1994.

WEANING CRITERIA

- Symptoms of pathological process are controlled
  - afebrile
  - chest X-ray clear
  - free of potentially lethal cardiac dysrhythmias
  - stable on medications (vasoactive drugs, etc.)
- Patient awake, alert enough to initiate spontaneous respirations
- Adequate natural airway or tracheostomy
- PaO_2 >60 mm Hg when receiving 40–60% O_2
- Able to mobilize secretions
- Spontaneous tidal volume (TV) >6 mL/kg
- Spontaneous vital capacity (VC) >15 mL/kg
- Inspiratory force ≥20 cm H_2O
- Compliance ≥20 mL/cm H_2O
- Acceptable ABG values
- Stable circulation

Discontinue weaning if
- **systolic B/P rises ≥20 mm Hg**
- **diastolic B/P rises ≥10 mm Hg**
- **increase in heart rate ≥20 beats/min**
- **heart rate >120 beats/min**
- **onset of dysrhythmia**
- **increase in respiratory rate ≥10 breaths/min**
- **respiratory rate >30 breaths/min**
- **labored breathing**
- **fatigue**
- **derangement of arterial blood gases**

EXTRACORPOREAL MEMBRANE OXYGENATION (ECMO)

An adaptation of cardiopulmonary bypass, ECMO involves the removal of deoxygenated blood, infusing it with oxygen, removing carbon dioxide, and returning the blood to systemic circulation. ECMO provides "resting" time, allowing the lungs to heal, but should be utilized only after other methods of oxygenation have failed.

Criteria
- PaO_2 level below 50 mm Hg with optimal PEEP for at least 2 hr
- Alveolar-arterial (A-a) oxygen difference at least 600 mm Hg
- Thirty percent of blood passing through lungs is unoxygenated

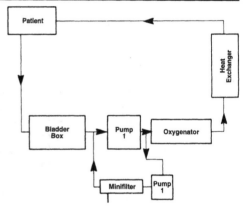

Figure 2.6 Extracorporeal Membrane Oxygenation
Reprinted with permission of Amicon Division of W.R. Grace & Co., Beverly, MA.

Method

Venovenous
- Large-bore cannula placed in saphenous, common iliac, or femoral vein
- Heart provides perfusion pressure and oxygenated blood is returned to the system *before* it enters the pulmonary circulation

Procedure
- Venous blood drained by gravity
- Blood collected in a bladder (collapsible) reservoir
- Blood circulated via roller pump through membrane oxygenator

Indications
- *Venovenous* ECMO has proven useful in *adult* patients
- Used for those patients suffering severe hypoxia of potentially reversible disorders
  – ARDS
  – pulmonary embolus

Method

Procedure

- Oxygenated blood passes through heat exchanger to maintain normothermia

Indications

- bacterial/viral pneumonia
- inhalation injuries
- Irreversible end-stage lung disease awaiting single lung or heart–lung transplant

Venoarterial

- Venous catheter caries blood to ECMO system; blood returned via an artery bypassing heart

- Blood removed through venous access catheter
- Pumped through membrane oxygenator
- Passes through heat exchanger to maintain temperature
- Returned to systemic circulation through arterial cannula

- *Venoarterial* ECMO most useful in treatment of *pediatric* patients
- Used for patients suffering severe hypoxia related to potentially reversible disorders
  - persistent fetal circulation
  - hyaline membrane disease
  - meconium aspiration
  - congenital heart defects
- Irreversible end-stage lung disease awaiting single lung or heart–lung transplant

Contraindications

- Pulmonary fibrosis
- Multiple organ failure
- CNS damage
- Cranial bleeding
- Irreversible shock
- Risk of bleeding
- Significant left heart failure

Complications

- Hemorrhage
- Thrombus formation
- Sepsis
- Cannula dislodgment
- Acute bleeding episodes
- Renal failure
- Fluid and electrolyte imbalance

Nursing/Medical Implications

- Requires specially trained personnel: perfusionist or ECMO technician
- Specialized equipment required; costly
- Patients may remain on system for several days
- Heparinization required; activated clotting time should be maintained at 200–240 sec (normal: <180 sec)

chapter 3

NEUROLOGICAL EVALUATION

EVALUATION OF CRANIAL NERVES

Nerve	Function	Assessment

I Olfactory
(Sensory)
	• Smell	• Have patient close eyes
		• Close off one nostril
		• Have patient identify nonirritating odors
		  – coffee
		  – cinnamon
		  – peppermint
		• Repeat process for other nostril

II Optic *(Sensory)*	• Vision	• Have patient count fingers • Assess light perception • Assess blink reflex • Use opthalmoscope for funduscopic examination

III Oculomotor
(Motor)
	• Constriction of pupils
	• Elevation of upper eyelid
	• Most movements of the eye
		• Test these nerves together, as functions overlap somewhat
		• Oculomotor
		  – compare size, shape of pupils
		  – compare pupillary response to light
		  – check for ptosis

IV Trochlear *(Motor)*	• Downward and inward movement of eye	

V Trigeminal
(Motor/sensory)
	• Ophthalmic branch—sensation to corneas, nasal mucosa, oral mucosa, facial skin
	• Maxillary and mandibular branch—strength of muscles of mastication
		• Facial sensory response
		  – stroke forehead with pin or wisp of cotton
		• Corneal reflex
		  – lightly touch cornea with wisp of cotton (reflex may be less in patients wearing contacts)
		  – avoid repeating test; highly irritating

		• Maxillary and mandibular
		  – have patient clench jaws tightly; attempt to pry open jaws with your fingers
		  – test for jaw jerk by having patient hold mouth slightly open; tap chin with reflex hammer; mouth should jerk closed

VI Abducens
(Motor)
	• Lateral movement of eye	• Oculomotor nerve passes through tentorium and is best indicator of herniation; a fixed dilated pupil occurs, usually on same side as herniation
		• Trochlear and abducens
		  – assess for conjugate and lateral eye movement
		• Check for Doll's eyes reflex to determine absence of injury to cervical spine
		  – when head is rotated in one direction, eyes normally move in opposite direction
		
		Pathological response would be that the eyes remain in the midline position when the head is rotated.

VII Facial **(Sensory/motor)**	• Control of facial muscles • Taste perception of anterior two thirds of tongue	• Upper and lower facial motor function – assess for facial symmetry at rest and when grimacing – have patient raise eyebrows, wrinkle forehead, puff out cheeks, show teeth

Nerve	Function	Assessment
VII Facial (cont.)		• Taste perception – place salty, sweet, sour, or bitter substances on tip of tongue (sugar, salt, or vinegar may be used)
VIII Acoustic (Sensory)	• Controls hearing (cochlear) • Controls equilibrium (vestibular)	• Hearing – ask patient to identify common sounds (snapping fingers, clock ticking, whisper) – use tuning fork to evaluate air and bone conduction • Equilibrium – in the critical care setting it may be impossible to assess equilibrium. Under ordinary circumstances the patient may be asked to maintain balance while standing with feet together, eyes closed and arms outstretched (ROMBERG TEST)
IX Glossopharyngeal (Motor/sensory)	• Controls ability to swallow and utter sound • Controls perception of taste on posterior one-third of tongue • Sensation of soft palate, pharyngeal, tonsillar mucosa • Salivation	• Closely related functionally and anatomically, glossopharyngeal and vagus nerves should be assessed together • Glossopharyngeal – test gag reflex by touching tongue depressor to patient's pharynx – have patient identify taste at back of tongue (salty/sweet discrimination)

X Vagus *(Motor/sensory)*	• Controls ability to swallow, utter sound
	• Sensation to outer ear (posterior wall) and behind ear
	• Sensation to abdominal, thoracic viscera
		• Vagus
		  – observe swallowing ability
		  – have patient say "ah" while observing soft palate for symmetry

XI Spinal *Accessory* *(Motor)*	• Controls movement of uvula, soft palate • Controls shoulder movement, neck rotation (trapezius) • Sternocleidomastoid muscle	• Have patient resist attempt to rotate head from one side to midline • Have patient shrug shoulders against resistance • Have patient stretch out hands
		None of these tests should be attempted until cervical spine injury has been ruled out.
XII Hypoglossal *(Motor)*	• Controls movement of tongue involved in swallowing, speaking	• Have patient stick out tongue; observe for tremor, asymmetry, deviation to one side, or fasciculation • To test for strength have patient move tongue against resistance

EVALUATION OF SEIZURE ACTIVITY

A primary seizure is referred to as a seizure with no identifiable cause. Secondary seizure results from identifiable causes such as congenital anomalies, tumors, head trauma, or cerebral vascular disease.

Phase	Symptoms	Duration	Nursing/Medical Implications

Prodromal	• Mood, behavior changes
	• Aura
	  – metallic taste
	  – unusual smell
	  – extraordinary sound
	  – flash of light or spots before eyes
		• May precede seizure by hours or days	• Nature of the aura may facilitate identification of seizure origin

Ictal	• Muscle spasms • Constriction of throat muscles • Apnea • Cyanosis • Hyperventilation • Tongue, lip biting • Bowel, bladder incontinence • Salivation	• Usually 2–5 min	• Scream or cry may immediately precede onset of activity • During this phase, patient may aspirate vomitus, occlude airway, or injure self
Postictal	• Lethargy • Confusion/disorientation • Fatigue • Headache • Memory loss • Irritability • Muscle weakness	• May last several hours	

DIFFERENTIATING SEIZURE ACTIVITY

PARTIAL/SIMPLE SEIZURES

Type	Clinical Manifestations	Level of Consciousness
Focal motor	• Convulsive movement in a body part controlled by a specific area of the brain	• Involvement of one hemisphere: no loss of consciousness • Involvement of both hemispheres: loss of consciousness
Focal sensory	• Subjective sensory occurrence; auditory, olfactory, visual, or somatosensory	• No change in consciousness level
Jacksonian	• Disturbance in motor activity, beginning at the peripheral part of a limb and extending to the proximal muscles; may extend to entire side and may become a generalized seizure	• One hemisphere: no change in level of consciousness • Both hemispheres: loss of consciousness
Adversive	• Head and eyes deviate from focal region • Disturbance in behavior/motor activity • May become generalized	• No loss of consciousness

Psychomotor
(Complex partial seizure)
	• Multiple sensory, motor, or psychic components
	  – outburst of temper
	  – anger
	  – fear
	  – automatisms
	  – hallucinations
		• May lose consciousness
		• May be unaware of event

GENERALIZED SEIZURES

Type	Clinical Manifestations	Level of Consciousness
Tonic–clonic *(Grand mal)*	• Major tonic muscular contractions • Longer clonic contractions • Bowel, bladder incontinence • Postictal weakness • Possible injury	• Loss of consciousness • Postictal somnolence
Absence *(Petit mal)*	• Paroxysmal attacks of impaired consciousness • Spasm or twitching of cephalic muscles	• Transient loss of consciousness • No postictal sequelae
Myoclonic	• Uncontrolled jerking movements of the extremities • May involve entire body	• Momentary loss of consciousness • Confusion
Akinetic *(Drop attack)*	• Epileptic manifestations (aura, extraordinary sound, smell, taste) without movement • Precipitous loss of postural tone	• No loss of consciousness • No postictal sequelae

ASSESSING BRAINSTEM FUNCTION USING THE DERM MNEMONIC

The Brainstem	Herniation Levels	D = Depth of Coma	E = Eyes	R = Respirations	M = Motor Function	Posturing
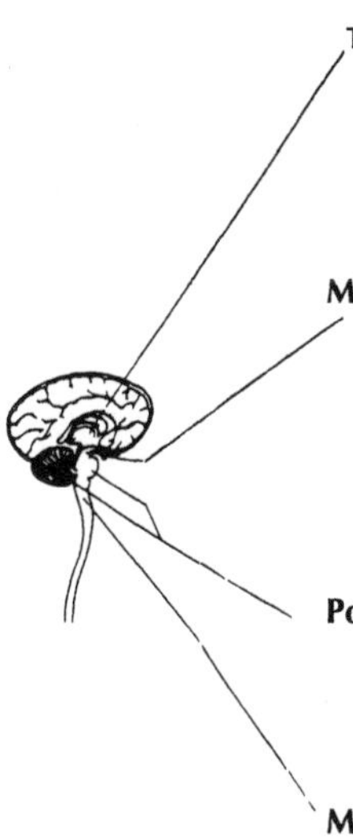	Thalmus	Painful stimulus causes nonpurposeful response	Pupils small; react to light	Eupnea 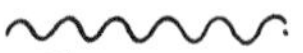 ∿∿∿∿∿ Cheyne–Stokes respirations 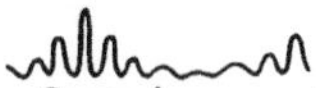 ᴡᴧᴧᴧ	Hyperactive deep tendon reflexes	Decorticate
	Midbrain	Painful stimulus causes no response	Midpoint to dilated; fixed; no reaction to light	Central neurogenic breathing 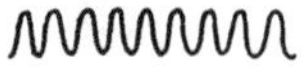 �ᴧᴧᴧᴧᴧᴧ	Decreased deep tendon reflexes	Decere-brate
	Pons	Painful stimulus causes no response	Midpoint to dilated; fixed; no reaction to light	Biot's respirations 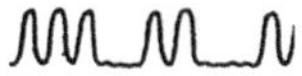 ᴧᴧᴧ_ᴧᴧ_ᴧ	Flaccid	No tone
	Medulla	Painful stimulus causes no response	Midpoint to dilated; fixed; no reaction to light	Ataxic/ apneustic 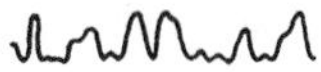 ᴧᴧᴧᴧᴧ	Flaccid	No tone

Reprinted with permission from Budassi, SA, and Barber, J: Mosby's Manual of Emergency Care, 2nd ed. St. Louis: CV Mosby, 1984.

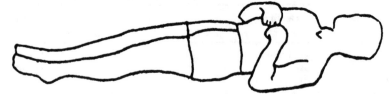

Figure 3.1   Decorticate: Arms Flexed at the Elbow and Hands Pulled Toward Midchest, Indicating a Lesion Above the Midbrain

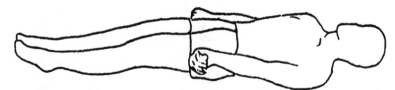

Figure 3.2   Decerebrate: Arms Extended and Hands Clenched, Rotated Outward, Indicating a Lesion at the Level of the Brainstem

MOTOR FUNCTION OF THE SPINAL CORD

A spinal cord injury above the T_2 level manifests as quadriplegia. Below T_2 it manifests as paraplegia.

Spinal Segment	Muscle	Function
C_2	• All muscles below trapezius • Sternocleidomastoid	• All movement except shoulder lift and head turning
$C_{3,4,5}$	• Diaphragm • Muscles of respiration	• Diaphragm excursion
C_5	• Trapezius	• Shoulder shrug
$C_{5,6}$	• Deltoids • Biceps • Extensor, carpi radialis	• Arm elevation • Elbow flexion • Wrist extension
$C_{6,7,8}$	• Triceps • Extensor digitorum	• Forearm extension • Finger extension
$C_{7,8}$	• Flexor carpi radialis • Flexor digitorum	• Wrist flexion • Finger grip
T_1	• Interossei	• Finger spreading
T_1–T_{12}	• Intercostals • Rectus abdominus/obliques	• Respiration • Trunk stability
$T_{11,12}$	• Levator ani • Detrusor • Bulbocavernosus/ischiocavernosus	• Voluntary bowel control • Voluntary bladder control • Achieving and maintaining an erection
$L_{1,2,3}$	• Iliopsoas	• Hip flexion
$L_{2,3,4}$	• Quadriceps, femoris	• Knee extension
L_4–S_2	• Biceps, femoris, hamstring • Extensor hallucis/digitorum	• Knee flexion • Foot dorsiflexion
L_5–S_2	• Gluteus maximus • Gastrocnemius	• Hip extension • Plantar flexion

GLASGOW COMA SCALE

The Glasgow Coma Scale is a reliable, objective instrument for evaluating level of consciousness. A cumulative score of 7 or less indicates that the patient is in a coma. Use of this tool obviates the use of ambiguous terms, such as stuporous, lethargic, or obtunded, when documenting level of consciousness.

Parameter	Score	Response
Eye opening	4	• Eyes open spontaneously
Determine *minimal* stimulus that evokes	3	• Eyes open in response to verbal stimulus
response	2	• Eyes open to painful stimulus
	1	• Eyes *do not* open even in response to pain
Verbal response	5	• Oriented to person, place and time; converses appropriately
Determine response after patient is aroused	4	• Converses but is confused
	3	• Uses inappropriate words and phrases
	2	• Sounds are incomprehensible
	1	• No verbal sound even in response to painful stimuli
Motor response	6	• Obeys verbal commands
Determine best response of either extremity	5	• Localizes and attempts to remove painful stimulus
	4	• Responds with flexion and withdrawal from painful stimulus
	3	• Abnormal flexion (decorticate posturing) in response to pain

TESTING FOR CEREBROSPINAL FLUID (CSF) LEAKAGE

- Any suspected CSF drainage may be tested with Dextrostix or Tes-Tape; CSF tests positive for glucose
- Another test for CSF leakage is known as the "halo" or "target" sign; observe suspected stains on bedding or on a paper or cloth; when CSF contains blood, the blood aggregates at the center and clear CSF dissipates outward, forming a halo
- Patient may complain of a salty taste in mouth from salt in the CSF

If CSF leakage is suspected, never suction or pack the nose or ears.

chapter 4

DIALYTIC THERAPY

Dialytic therapy is performed for removal of excess water, correction of electrolyte imbalance, correction of acid-base disturbances, and removal of waste matter, drugs, and toxins. Dialysis is based on the principles of diffusion, osmosis, and ultrafiltration. Before insertion, utilization, or management of any dialysis device, refer to manufacturer's product information.

HEMODIALYSIS

Hemodialysis is the movement of toxified blood from the artery to the dialyzer and back to the venous circulation. The blood is heparinized, passed through the dialyzer, detoxified, and returned to the circulation (see Figure 4.1).

The dialysis process is managed by a specially trained hemodialysis nurse. However, the patient remains the responsibility of assigned personnel pre- and postdialysis.

Indications
- Renal failure
  - critical volume excess
  - respiratory insufficiency
  - electrolyte disturbances, particularly hyperkalemia
  - abdominal wall deformity that precludes peritoneal dialysis
  - when dialysis must be accomplished quickly

Contraindications
- Severe blood dyscrasia
- Cardiovascular disease
- Atherosclerosis
- Unavailable vascular access sites
- Shock or hypotension
- Religious opposition to hemodialysis

Components

- Kidney (dialyzer) has a blood compartment, a dialysate compartment, and a semipermeable membrane. Water, electrolytes, and small molecules of waste product pass through this membrane. Larger elements, such as protein, RBCs, and bacteria, are too large to pass through the membrane
- The dialysate is an electrolyte solution much like normal plasma; potassium concentrations vary according to patient need. Although glucose is a large molecule, it can pass through the semipermeable membrane; therefore glucose may be added to the dialysate to maintain serum glucose and osmolality

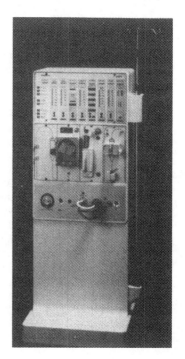

Figure 4.1 Hemodialysis Machine

Reprinted with permission of Fresenius USA, Inc. (2637 Shadelands Drive, Walnut Creek, CA 94598), 1995.

- Vascular access
  - internal AV fistula: surgical connection of vein and artery; allows normal arterial blood pressure to pump blood; has minimal clotting and infection risk; allows unrestricted movement of the involved extremity; may cause parasthesias below the fistula site; not usable if patient's veins are small
  - autogenous saphenous vein graft, bovine graft, umbilical cord graft, synthetic (dacron) graft: allows arterial blood pressure to pump blood; may be inserted in arm or thigh; permits unrestricted movement of the involved extremity; may clot off in the presence of hypotension; tissue surrounding graft may become infected
  - femoral vein catheterization: quick, emergency access, with double- or single-lumen catheter; requires immobilization of patient; carries risk of thrombus, femoral artery trauma, and site infection; should not be in place >2–4 days
  - subclavian vein catheterization: quick, emergency access, facilitates patient movement; less apt than femoral access to become infected; high risk of pneumothorax; contraindicated in patient with pulmonary hypertension; manufacturer recommends removal of catheter after 3 weeks of use

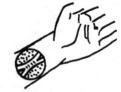

Figure 4.2A   AV Fistula

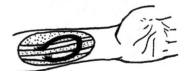

Figure 4.2B   Vein Graft—Arteriovenous Graft

- arteriovenous (AV) shunt: a surgically created anastomosis of an artery and a vein; allows arterial blood pressure to pump blood from artery to vein via an external silastic tube; decreases need for repeated venipuncture/cannulation; carries clotting and infection risk; restricts movement of the involved extremity. *Greatest risk* is hemorrhage and death if apparatus separates; two clamps should always be kept readily available in case of cannulae disconnect
- hemasite: T-shaped device placed into an arterialized vein via a dacron graft; provides T-shaped external entry site

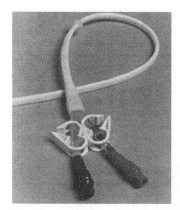

Figure 4.2C   Quinton PermCath Catheter

Reprinted with permission of Quinton Instrument Co. (Bothell, WA), 1995.

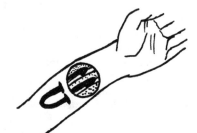

Figure 4.2D   AV Shunt

Nursing/Medical Implications
- As an internal fistula matures, the vein becomes arterialized, enhancing high blood flow pressure; fistula requires 4–6 weeks for maturity
- Fistula patency can be determined by auscultation for a bruit or palpating for a thrill; other signs of occluded access are cold, clammy, pulseless, cynotic extremity and evidence of serum separation in cannula (areas of clear serum or black clots in cannula)
- Monitor for arterial steal syndrome, particularly in arm; poor arterial flow may cause shunting of blood supply to fingers; signs of decreased arterial flow to fingers will be noted
- When connecting/disconnecting blood lines to catheter all care must be taken to prevent introduction of air into blood path
- Access site not recommended for routine blood drawing, but may be used if no other site is available; strict aseptic technique must be observed; must never be drawn from an immature fistula/graft <6 weeks old
- One-way obstruction may be caused by tip malposition; if lumen can be flushed but not aspirated, repositioning catheter may be necessary
- Patients receiving digitalis should be monitored closely for serum potassium levels
- Air embolism is a complication of hemodialysis; signs/symptoms are dyspnea, chest pain, confusion, coughing, visual problems, and ringing in ears; emergency treatment includes placing patient on left side with head lower than feet and administering oxygen
- Requires 3–5 hr to complete treatment
- Weigh patient pre- and postdialysis; order lab work as clinically indicated

INTERMITTENT PERITONEAL DIALYSIS (IPD)

Peritoneal dialysis differs from hemodialysis in that the patient's own peritoneum serves as the semipermeable membrane utilized to filter solutes and fluid. This technique is less efficient than hemodialysis but, in some instances, is better tolerated by patients unable to tolerate rapid fluid and electrolyte shifts. This technique can be managed by nursing staff without the intensive training required for hemodialysis. Some newer methods—continuous ambulatory peritoneal dialysis (CAPD) and continuous cyclic peritoneal dialysis (CCPD)—can be accomplished by the patient at home.

Indications
- Renal failure:
  – with blood clotting disorder precluding hemodialysis
  – cardiovascular disease
  – atherosclerosis
  – unavailable arterio/venous access sites
  – religious opposition to hemodialysis
- Patient able to manage dialysis at home
- Diabetic patient
- Patient suffering intractable hypotension as a result of hemodialysis
- Malignant hypertension
- Severe anemia requiring transfusions

Contraindications
- Abdominal deformities, such as surgery, draining abdominal wounds, abdominal wall infection, or severe intra-abdominal adhesions
- Patient undergoing immunosuppressive therapy
- Patient with chronic obstructive pulmonary disease
- Poor peritoneal clearance
- Organomegaly
- Profound obesity

Components
- Catheter
  - trocar; a stiff silastic catheter
  - soft silastic indwelling catheter
- Dialysate
  - a sterile electrolyte solution similar to normal plasma; ionized calcium used to maintain positive calcium balance, as patients in renal failure tend to be hypocalcemic; glucose concentrations vary—hypertonic solutions increase osmotic pressure, and consequent filtration clearance; potassium concentrations vary according to patient need
- Abdominal access
  - below umbilicus
- Catheter
  - may be temporary or permanent
  - a trocar; a stiff silastic catheter that may be inserted at the bedside
  - indwelling catheter; soft silastic device inserted in surgery
  - tip terminates in the true pelvis or vesicorectal fossa

Phases of Dialysis
- Inflow phase
  - time involved in instilling the dialysate in the peritoneal cavity; may vary, depending on volume and patient response
- Dwell time (diffusion phase)
  - time that dialysate remains in peritoneal cavity; varies with patient's clinical response
- Outflow phase
  - time required to drain dialysate from peritoneal cavity, along with any excess fluid

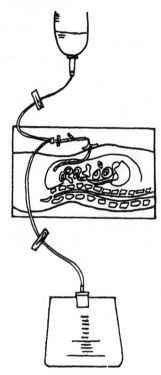

Figure 4.3 Peritoneal Dialysis

Nursing/Medical Implications
- Assess for bowel or urinary bladder distention; distention increases risk of perforation
- Strict aseptic technique is imperative; peritonitis is most serious complication of peritoneal dialysis
- Amount of fluid drained from the cavity should be greater than amount instilled
- Fluid balance should be calculated at end of each exchange
- Monitor patient response, particularly discomfort, respiratory distress, signs/ symptoms of fluid and electrolyte imbalance
- Complications include
  - perforation of bowel, bladder, or viscera
  - hemorrhage
  - peritonitis
  - dehydration
  - fluid and electrolyte imbalances
  - hyperglycemia
  - cardiac dysrhythmias
  - catheter occlusion
- Dialysate should be warmed prior to use to minimize body heat loss
- Monitor abdominal girth as an indicator of dialysate retention
- Monitor catheter site for bleeding or fluid leakage
- Air trapped in dialysate may impede adequate outflow

CONTINUOUS ARTERIOVENOUS HEMOFILTRATION (CAVH)

CAVH is a means of reducing fluid overload without potential complications inherent in hemodialysis. This technique removes plasma, water, and dissolved solutes from the intravascular fluid but allows conservation of cellular and protein components.

CAVH is an uncomplicated procedure and does not require specialized management. The determinants involved are hydrostatic pressure, blood flow, oncotic pressure, pericapillary pressure, and ultrafiltration coefficient.

Indications
- Refractory fluid overload/CHF
- Inadequate renal function
- Poor response to diuretics or vasodilators
- Coagulopathy
- Abdominal deformities that limit use of peritoneal dialysis
- Patients on parenteral nutrition requiring fluid restriction
- Hypercatabolic/hyperosmolar states
- Unstable hemodynamic status
- Multiple organ failure

Contraindications
- Hypotension
- Need for *rapid* removal of fluids/solutes

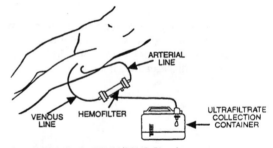

Figure 4.4 Basic CAVH/SCUF Circuit
Reprinted with permission of Minntech Corp. (14605 28th Avenue North, Minneapolis, MN 55447), 1995.

Components
- Hemofiltration device
  - cylinder containing bundles of hollow fibers or capillaries that act as semipermeable membranes
  - arterial line that moves blood from patient to filter; must be large enough to allow unobstructed blood flow
  - venous line that moves blood from filter back to vascular circulation
- Infusion pump to control rate of heparin infusion, concomitant IV fluids, filtration replacement fluid, parenteral nutrition, etc.
- Ultrafiltration collection bag with measuring graduate
- Access
  - internal AV fistula
  - arteriovenous shunt/graft
  - femoral/subclavian vein catheterization

Nursing/Medical Implications
- Force of gravity and patient's B/P power CAVH
- As blood pressure drops, so does filtration
- Ultrafiltrate should be removed at a rate of *at least* 8 cc/min
- Slow rate of hemofiltration reduces risk of hypotension and dramatic fluid and electrolyte shift
- Hemofiltration is a continuous process; used for limited periods of time
- Requires no complex equipment
- With CAVH, less blood circulates extracorporeally and less heparin is required to prevent clotting
- Complications include
  - bleeding
  - volume depletion
  - air embolism
  - cardiac dysrhythmias
  - acidosis

- infection
- clogged lines
- Rate of ultrafiltration is adjusted according to patient response to fluid removal as indicated by body weight, B/P, central venous pressure, and pulmonary artery pressure
- Ultrafiltrate rate is regulated by position of collection chamber; negative hydrostatic pressure increases as chamber is lowered
- Filter and lines should be placed close to access extremity

SLOW CONTINUOUS ULTRAFILTRATION (SCUF)

SCUF is indicated in the prevention and treatment of overhydration in oliguric and anuric patients, while adequate amounts of intravenous infusions and parenteral nutrition are maintained.

Indications
- Relief of fluid overload
- "Making space" for IV infusions
- In some cases continuous hemofiltration may be carried out with little or no heparin in patients considered risky for bleeding

Contraindications
- Need for removal of uremic toxins

Components
- Setup for SCUF is essentially the same as that for CAVH; major difference between the two is degree of filtration; the terms, in some cases, may be used interchangeably

Nursing/Medical Implications
- Rate of ultrafiltrate removal should keep pace with fluid intake (i.e., IV solutions, hyperalimentation)

CONTINUOUS ARTERIOVENOUS HEMODIAFILTRATION (CAVH-D)

CAVH-D enhances the clearance of low-molecular-weight solutes and combines the advantages of continuous hemofiltration and the clearance capabilities of hemodialysis.

Sterile dialysate flows counter to the direction of blood flow into the side port at the venous end of the unit and out of the side port at the arterial end. The dialysate provides a concentration gradient that allows selective removal of large amounts of uremic solutes.

The procedure may be simplified by decreasing the ultrafiltration rate to <5 mL/min, obviating the need for replacement fluid. The primary principle involved is diffusion.

Indications
- Need for high rates of low molecular weight solute clearances not achievable with standard CAVH alone
  - acute catabolic renal failure
  - hypervolemia
  - uremia

Components
- Same as for CAVH with addition of
  - dialysate, which enters hemofilter at venous end and exits, along with ultrafiltrate, at arterial end

Nursing/Medical Implications
- Same as with CAVH

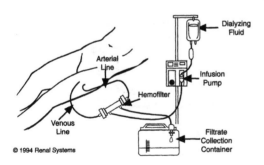

© 1994 Renal Systems

Figure 4.5   CAVH-D (hemodiafiltration) Countercurrent Flow
Reprinted with permission of Minntech Corp. (Minneapolis), 1995.

CONTINUOUS VENOUS–VENOUS HEMOFILTRATION (CVVH)

CVVH is performed when arterial access is inappropriate or impossible. Access is obtained by means of double-lumen venous catheter or separate venous cannulae utilizing the subclavian vein or via an AV fistula. A blood pump is attached to the extracorporeal circuit. The rate of blood flow should be approximately 100 mL/min.

Use of the blood pump indicates the need for specially trained nursing personnel at bedside to prevent disconnection and exsanguination.

Indications
• Unavailable arterial access

Components
• Hemofiltration device (hemofilter) same as that used for CAVH and CAVH-D
• Double-lumen catheter or separate venous cannulae
• Blood pump to maintain adequate flow through system
• Substitution fluid attached to blood outflow line

Nursing/Medical Implications
• Same as CAVH/CAVH-D

CVVH-D is CVVH with the addition of sterile dialysis solution infused countercurrent to the blood flow— HEMODIAFILTRATION.

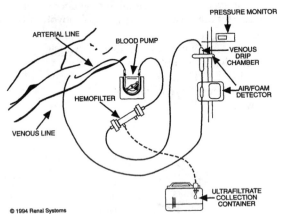

© 1994 Renal Systems

Figure 4.6A   CVVH Pump-Assisted Circuit

Reprinted with permission of Minntech Corp. (Minneapolis), 1995.

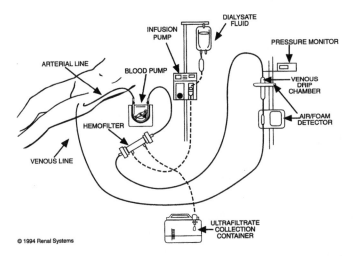

DIALYSATE
FLUID

INFUSION
PUMP

PRESSURE MONITOR

ARTERIAL LINE

BLOOD PUMP

VENOUS
DRIP
CHAMBER

HEMOFILTER

AIR/FOAM
DETECTOR

VENOUS LINE

© 1994 Renal Systems

ULTRAFILTRATE
COLLECTION
CONTAINER

Figure 4.6B CVVH-D

Reprinted with permission of Minntech Corp.
(Minneapolis), 1995.

chapter 5

IV FLUIDS

DEXTROSE SOLUTIONS

Solution	pH	Elemental Composition	Therapeutic Value	Nursing Implications/Precautions	Access
$D_{2.5}W$ (Hypotonic)	4.0–5.1	• Calories (85)	• Maintains water balance/prevents dehydration • Supplies calories • Maintains blood sugar • Prevents/treats ketosis	• Not for use in blood administration • May intensify hypokalemia • Possible fluid overload • Pulmonary congestion • Peripheral edema	• Peripheral vein
D_5W (Isotonic)	4.0–5.0	• Calories (170)	• Enhances renal excretion of solutes	• Serum glucose elevation • Hyperosmolar syndrome • Water intoxication	
$D_{10}W$ (Hypertonic)	4.0–4.6	• Calories (340)	• Peripheral nutrition • Provides calories in minimal water	• May worsen renal damage	
$D_{20}W$ (Hypertonic)	4.0–4.6	• Calories (680)	• Diuretic • Reduces CNS edema • TPN	• Peripheral vein irritation • May produce hypercalcemia, hypermagnesemia, hyperphosphatemia, hyperglycemia, hyperosmolar syndrome	• Large vein (femoral/jugular)
$D_{30}W$ $D_{40}W$ $D_{50}W$ $D_{60}W$ $D_{70}W$ (Hypertonic)	4.0–4.7 4.0–5.0	• Calories (1020) • Calories (1360) • Calories (1700) • Calories (2040) • Calories (2380)			• Central line

SALINE SOLUTIONS

Solution	pH	Elemental Composition	Therapeutic Value	Nursing Implications/Precautions	Access
0.45% NaCl (Hypotonic)	4.8–5.3	• Na$^+$ (77 mEq/L) • Cl$^-$ (77 mEq/L) • No calories	• Maintains hydration/ extracellular fluid volume • Expands plasma volume • Maintains serum sodium concentrations	• Use cautiously with patients suffering heart disease, renal disease, hepatic disease • May cause CHF/ pulmonary edema	• Peripheral vein
0.9% NaCl (Isotonic)	4.8–5.7	• Na$^+$ (154 mEq/L) • Cl$^-$ (154 mEq/L) • No calories	• Initiation and termination of blood transfusion • Regulates acid–base volume • Dehydration • Management of hyperosmolar diabetes	• Derangement of serum electrolyte concentration • Overhydration • Venous thrombosis • May cause hyperatremia • May cause peripheral edema	
3.0% NaCl (Hypertonic)	5.0–5.8	• Na$^+$ (513 mEq/L) • Cl$^-$ (513 mEq/L) • No calories	• Corrects significant sodium depletion • Diabetic coma • Addisonian crisis	• Administer hypertonic saline at slow rate	
5.0% NaCl (Hypertonic)	4.5–7.0	• Na$^+$ (855 mEq/L) • Cl$^-$ (855 mEq/L) • No calories	• Maximum daily amount not to exceed 400 mL		

DEXTROSE/SALINE SOLUTIONS

Solution	pH	Elemental Composition	Therapeutic Value	Nursing Implications/Precautions	Access
Dextrose 2.5% in NaCl 0.45% (Hypotonic)	4.0–4.6	• Na$^+$ (77 mEq/L) • Cl$^-$ (77 mEq/L) • Calories (85)	• Provides calories, salt, water	• CHF • Pulmonary edema • Sodium retention if patient has compromised renal function • Derangement of serum electrolyte concentrations • Overhydration	• Peripheral vein
Dextrose 5% in NaCl 0.45% (Hypotonic)	3.5–6.5	• Na$^+$ (77 mEq/L) • Cl$^-$ (77 mEq/L) • Calories (170)	• Treatment of hypovolemia • Promotes diuresis in dehydration		
Dextrose 5% in NaCl 0.9% (Hypertonic)	4.0–4.4	• Na$^+$ (154 mEq/L) • Cl$^-$ (154 mEq/L) • Calories (170)	• Same as above		

RINGER'S SOLUTIONS

Solution	pH	Elemental Composition	Therapeutic Value	Nursing Implications/Precautions	Access
Ringer's injection (Isotonic)	5.5–6.0	• Na^+ (147.5 mEq/L) • Cl^- (156 mEq/L) • Ca^{2+} (4.5 mEq/L) • K^+ (4 mEq/L)	• Replaces Na^+, Cl^-, Ca^{2+}, K^+ • Treats dehydration caused from reduced fluid intake, vomiting, diarrhea • Treatment of mild alkalosis • Treatment of hypochloremia • Burns	• Use cautiously in patients with CHF, severe renal insufficiency, or edema with sodium retention • Exercise care in administering to patients with hyperkalemia, hypercalcemia, renal failure, or potassium retention • May cause fluid and/or solute overload	• Peripheral vein
D_5R (Hypertonic)	4.0–4.6	• Na^+ (147.5 mEq/L) • Cl^- (156 mEq/L) • Ca^{2+} (4.5 mEq/L) • K^+ (4 mEq/L) • Calories (170)	• Same as above	• Overhydration • Congestive states • Pulmonary edema	

RINGER'S SOLUTIONS *continued*

Solution	pH	Elemental Composition	Therapeutic Value	Nursing Implications/Precautions	Access
Lactated Ringer's (Isotonic)	6.3–6.7	• Na$^+$ (130 mEq/L) • Cl$^-$ (109 mEq/L) • Ca^{2+} (3 mEq/L) • K$^+$ (4 mEq/L) • Lactate (28 mEq/L) • Calories (9)	• Replacement of Na$^+$, Cl$^-$, Ca^{2+}, K$^+$ • Correction of mild metabolic acidosis • Replacement of fluid loss caused by bile drainage, burns, diarrhea, acute blood loss	• Use with great care in patients with metabolic or respiratory alkalosis • Overhydration • Congestive states • Pulmonary edema • Excessive administration of lactate solution may result in metabolic alkalosis	• Peripheral vein
D$_5$LR (Hypertonic)	4.7–5.1	• Na$^+$ (130 mEq/L) • Cl$^-$ (109 mEq/L) • Ca^{2+} (3 mEq/L) • K$^+$ (4 mEq/L) • Lactate (28 mEq/L) • Calories (170–180)	• Same as above	• Same as above	

FAT EMULSIONS

Solution	pH	Elemental Composition	Therapeutic Value	Nursing Implications/Precautions	Access
Liposyn/intralipids 10% (Isotonic)	8.0	• Calories (1.1/mL) • Calories (1100/L)	• Concentrated source of calories • Parenteral nutrition requirement • Long-term nutritional support • Correction of fatty acid deficiency	• Chest pain (rare) • Thrombophlebitis • Thrombocytopenia **Indications are bleeding gums, nose bleeds, and hematuria.** • Anemia • Triglyceride elevation • Do not use filter • Infusion should not exceed 100 mL/hr	• Peripheral or central vein **Begin infusion at 1 mL/ min.**
Liposyn/intralipids 20% (Isotonic)	8.3	• Calories (2.0/mL) • Calories (2200/L)	• Same as above	• Should provide no more than 60% of total calorie intake • No drugs or solutions should be added to fat emulsions • May be administered simultaneously with amino acid solutions via Y-type infusion set • Should be administered through non-PVC administration set	**Begin infusion at 0.5 mL/ min.**

AMINO ACID SOLUTIONS

Amino acid solutions provide protein calories for anabolic purposes. The calories in these solutions should not be included in any calorie count because they *do not* provide energy/fuel to the catabolic patient. Energy calories should be provided solely by the addition of dextrose and lipids. The calories listed in these charts are *nonprotein* (dextrose) calories.

Solution	pH	N^{2+} (g/100 ml)	(mOsm/L)	Na^+ (mEq/L)	K^+ (mEq/L)	Ca^{2+} (mEq/L)	Mg^{2+} (mEq/L)	Cl^- (mEq/L)	Acetate (mEq/L)	PO_4 (mM/L)	Amino Acids
Aminosyn											
3.5%	5.3	0.55	357	7					46		3.5%
3.5% M	5.3	0.55	477	47	13		3	40	58	3.5	3.5%
5%	5.3	0.786	500		5.4				86		5%
7%	5.3	1.1	700		5.4				105	3.5	7%
7%	6.0	1.1	711		2.7				78		7%
7% with electrolytes	5.3	1.1	1013	70	66		10	96	124	30	7%
8.5%	5.3	1.34	850		5.4			35	90		8.5%
8.5%	6.0	1.34	856		2.7			11.7	90		8.5%
8.5% with electrolytes	5.3	1.34	1160	70	66		10	98	142	30	8.5%
10%	5.3	1.57	1000		5.4				148		10%
10%	6.0	1.57	993		2.7				111		10%
Aminosyn II											
3.5%	5.0–6.5	0.54	308	16.3					25.2		3.5%
3.5% M	5.0–6.5	0.54	425	36	13		3	37	25	3.5	3.5%
5%	5.0–6.5	0.77	438	19.3					35.9		5%

7%	5.0–6.5	1.07	612	31.3					50.3		7%
7% with electrolytes	5.0–6.5	1.07	869	80	66		10	86	50	30	7%
8.5%	5.0–6.5	1.30	742	33.3					61.1		8.5%
8.5% with electrolytes	5.0–6.5	1.30	999	84	66		10	86	61	30	8.5%
10%	5.0–6.5	1.53	873	45.3					71.8		10%
10% with electrolytes	5.0–6.5	1.53	1130	87	66		10	86	72	30	10%
FreAmine III											
3% with electrolytes	6.8	0.46	405	35	24.5		5	41	44	3.5	3%
8.5%	6.5	1.3	810	10				<3	72	10	8.5%
8.5% with electrolytes	6.0–7.0	1.3	1045	60	60		10	60	125	20	8.5%
10%	6.5	1.53	950	10				<3	89	10	10%
Travasol											
3.5% with electrolytes	6.0	0.591	450	25	15		5	25	52	7.5	3.5%
5.5%	6.0	0.925	575					22	48		5.5%
5.5% with electrolytes	6.0	0.925	850	70	60		10	70	102	30	5.5%
8.5%	6.0	1.43	890					34	73		8.5%

AMINO ACID SOLUTIONS *Continued*

Solution	pH	N^{2+} (g/100 ml)	(mOsm/L)	Na^+ (mEq/L)	K^+ (mEq/L)	Ca^{2+} (mEq/L)	Mg^{2+} (mEq/L)	Cl^- (mEq/L)	Acetate (mEq/L)	PO_4 (mM/L)	Amino Acids
8.5% with electrolytes	6.0	1.43	1160	70	60		10	70	141	30	8.5%
10%	6.0	1.65	1000					40	87		10%
Novamine 11.4%	5.6	1.8	1057						114		11.4%
15%	5.2–6.0	2.37	1388						151		15%
ProcalAmine (3% amino acid and 3% glycerin)	6.8	0.46	735	35	24	3	5	41	47	3.5	3%

PREMIX DEXTROSE/AMINO ACID SOLUTIONS

Solution	pH	Nonprotein (Kcal/L)	N²⁺ (g/100ml)	(mOsm/L)	Na⁺ (mEq/L)	K⁺ (mEq/L)	Ca²⁺ (mEq/L)	Mg²⁺ (mEq/L)	Cl⁻ (mEq/L)	Acetate (mEq/L)	PO₄ (mM/L)	Amino Acids
Aminosyn II												
3.5% and dextrose 5% (Nutrimix)	5.0–6.5	170	0.54	585	18					25.2		3.5%
3.5% and dextrose 25% (Nutrimix)	5.0–6.5	850	0.54	1515	18					25.2		3.5%
3.5% with electrolytes and dextrose 25% (Nutrimix)	5.0–6.5	850	0.54	1420	40	33		5	43	25.1	15	3.5%
3.5% M and dextrose 5% (Nutrimix)	5.0–6.5	170	0.54	616	41	13		3	36.5	25.1	3.5	3.5%
4.25% and dextrose 25% (Nutrimix)	5.0–6.5	850	0.65	1536	19					30.6		4.25%

PREMIX DEXTROSE/AMINO ACID SOLUTIONS   *Continued*

Solution	pH	Nonprotein (Kcal/L)	N^{2+} (g/100ml)	(mOsm/L)	Na$^+$ (mEq/L)	K$^+$ (mEq/L)	Ca^{2+} (mEq/L)	Mg^{2+} (mEq/L)	Cl$^-$ (mEq/L)	Acetate (mEq/L)	PO$_4$ (mM/L)	Amino Acids
4.25% with electrolytes and dextrose 25% (Nutrimix)	5.0–6.5	850	0.65	1438	42	33		5	43	30.5	15	4.25%
4.25% M and dextrose 10% (Nutrimix)	5.0–6.5	340	0.65	919	43.7	13		3	36.5	30.5	3.5	4.25%
5% and dextrose 25% (Nutrimix)	5.0–6.5	850	0.77	1539	22.2					35.9		5%

Indications
- Prevention of negative nitrogen balance in patients unable to take adequate nutrition by mouth
- Treatment of poor nutritional status resulting from hypermetabolic states, malabsorption syndrome, or chronic illness
- Conditions that require complete bowel rest over a period of time (ulcerative colitis, Crohn's disease, etc.)

Contraindications
- Hepatic or renal disease; specialized solutions available for such patients
- Metabolic disorders related to impaired nitrogen utilization
- Hypersensitivity to amino acids
- Patients prone to circulatory overload, particularly those with cardiac insufficiency

Nursing/Medical Implications
- TPN solutions must be infused at steady rate; do not attempt to "catch up" if infusion falls behind; severe metabolic shifts may result
- If TPN solution unavailable, continue with dextrose 10% to maintain venous access; abrupt cessation of TPN may result in rebound hypoglycemia; discontinue TPN gradually
- Patients, generally, spill 2+ urine glucose for the first 48 hr of TPN administration; pancreas adjusts to high glucose load in about 2 days; monitor blood glucose levels every 4–6 hr
- Do not use TPN line for drawing or giving blood, piggybacking other solutions, or administering medications
- Filter may be used according to hospital policy
- Single bottle of TPN solution should not hang for more than 24 hr
- Do not mix medications other than insulin with TPN; consult pharmacist as necessary
- Infusion rate should not exceed 4 mg/kg of nitrogen per hour
- Constantly observe infusion site for fever, erythema, phlebitis, and thrombosis
- Carefully monitor fluid intake, especially in patients with cardiac insufficiency
- Administration of amino acids may outstrip liver function; blood ammonia levels may rise to undesirable levels
- Metabolic acidosis has been seen with various amino acid solutions
- Monitor ammonia level and acid-base status closely

RENAL FORMULA

Solution	pH	N^{2+} (g/100mL)	(mOsm/L)	Na^+ (mEq/L)	K^+ (mEq/L)	Ca^{2+} 1(mEq/L)	Mg^{2+} (mEq/L)	Cl^- (mEq/L)	Acetate (mEq/L)	PO_4 (mM/L)	Amino Acids
Aminess 5.2%	6.4	0.66	416						50		5.2%
Aminosyn RF 5.2%	5.2	0.787	475		5.4				105		5.2%
NephrAmine 5.4%	6.5	0.64	435	5				<3	44		5.4%
RenAmine 6.5%	6.0	1.0	600					31	60		6.5%

Indications
- Prevention of negative nitrogen balance in patients unable to take adequate nutrition by mouth and suffering some form of renal disease

Treatment indicated particularly for patients experiencing renal failure or uremia and patients undergoing hemo/peritoneal dialysis.

Contraindications
- Uncorrected electrolyte or acid–base imbalance
- Hyperammonemia
- Decreased circulating blood volume
- Persons displaying symptoms of allergy to sulfite
- Potential for circulatory overload, particularly patients with cardiac insufficiency

Nursing/Medical Implications

- Azotemic patient should receive adequate protein to maximize protein utilization and minimize urea production
- For patients undergoing frequent hemo/peritoneal dialysis, 1.5–2.0 L of amino acid solutions (renal) should be administered daily
- High concentrations of dextrose (50–70%) should provide 2000 Kcal/day
- Fat emulsions may be used judiciously to augment calories provided by amino acid solutions
- Histidine and arginine reduce possibility of hyperammonemia
- Amino acids increase BUN concentrations; if renal function is inadequate, BUN will be elevated
- Uremic patient is frequently glucose intolerant, especially when undergoing peritoneal dialysis; exogenous insulin may be required to prevent hyperglycemia
- Patients intolerant to K^+ or Na^+ may require specific electrolyte solutions
- Refer to nursing implications for amino acid solutions on p. 211

HEPATIC FORMULA

Solution	pH	N^{2+} (g/100mL)	(mOsm/L)	Na^+ (mEq/L)	K^+ (mEq/L)	Ca^{2+} (mEq/L)	Mg^{2+} (mEq/L)	Cl^- (mEq/L)	Acetate (mEq/L)	PO_4 (mM/L)	Amino Acids
Aminosyn											
HBC 7%	5.2	1.12	665	7				≤40	72		7%
BranchAmine	6.0	0.443	316								4%
FreAmine											
6.9% HBC	6.5	0.97	620					<3	57		6.9%
HepatAmine	6.5	1.2	785					<3	62	10	8%

Indications
- Patients who require parenteral nutrition and because of hepatic encephalopathy are intolerant of general purpose amino acid solutions

Treatment indicated particularly for patients with hepatic failure, cirrhosis, and hepatitis.

Contraindications
- In hepatic failure, hepatic coma may be induced by accumulation of nitrogenous wastes; amino acid solutions may increase nitrogenous material accumulation
- Potential for circulatory overload, particularly patients with cardiac insufficiency

Nursing/Medical Implications
- For the moderately catabolic, depleted patient, in whom central venous route is not indicated, FreAmine HBC, Aminosyn–HBC 7% or HepatAmine may be diluted with 5–10% dextrose and infused by peripheral vein; supplemental fat emulsion also may be included
- Total daily intake of amino acid solutions/hepatic formula is 2–3 L; patients on fluid restriction may tolerate only 1–2 L
- Nitrogen or glucose intolerance or fluid restriction may preclude supplying higher nitrogen requirements in severely hypercatabolic or depleted patients
- Patients intolerant of K^+ or Na^+ may require specific electrolyte solutions
- Refer to nursing implications for amino acid solutions on p. 211

MONITORING THE PATIENT ON AMINO ACID SOLUTIONS

Variable to Be Monitored	Frequency	
	First Week	*Subsequently*
Height	At initiation of therapy	
Weight	Daily	Daily
Temperature/apical pulse/blood pressure/respirations	Daily	Daily
Anthropometric measurements	At initiation of therapy	Every 3 weeks
Volume of infusate	Daily	Daily
Oral intake (if any)	Daily	Daily
Urinary output, ostomy output, fistula, NG, etc.	Daily	Daily
Hgb/Hct/WBC/differential	Once	Weekly
Platelet count	Twice	prn
Total lymphocyte	Initially	Monthly
Serum electrolytes (Na^+, K^+, Cl^-, CO_2)	Daily	Twice weekly
BUN	Three times	Weekly
Creatinine, Ca^{2+}, PO_4, Mg^{2+}, total protein, albumin	2–3 times	Weekly
Blood glucose	Twice daily for first 2 days, then daily for 5 days	Twice weekly
PT, PTT	Twice	Weekly
Cholesterol, triglyceride	Twice	Weekly
Fe, TIBC, transferrin	Once	prn
Liver enzymes: SGOT, LDH, alk. phos., bilirubin D/T	Twice	Weekly
Ammonia	Three times	As clinically indicated
Cultures	As clinically indicated	As clinically indicated

This suggested schedule is for obtaining lab work for those patients receiving TPN. Institutional policies and procedures may vary and should be followed.

MONITORING THE PATIENT ON SPECIALIZED SOLUTIONS

In addition to the initial lab work, the patient on hepatic or renal solutions should be monitored for the following variables.

Variable to Be Monitored	Frequency	
	First Week	*Subsequently*
BUN	Daily	Twice weekly
Urea nitrogen appearance	Three times	Weekly
Blood ammonia	Once	As clinically indicated
Creatinine/urea clearance if GFR > 2 mL/min	Once	Weekly

CALCULATING CALORIE NEEDS

HARRIS–BENEDICT EQUATION[†]

$$BEE = 66.5 + 13.7W + 5.0H - 6.8A \quad \text{(male)}$$
$$BEE = 65.5 + 9.6W + 1.7H - 4.7A \quad \text{(female)}$$

CALVIN LONG—ACTIVITY FACTOR

1. Calculate the increased energy expenditure imposed by activity
   a. BEE × activity factor = REE
      (1) Confined to bed—1.2
      (2) Out of bed—1.3
2. Calculate the increased energy expenditure imposed by injury
   a. BEE × activity × injury = total estimation of energy requirements (TEE)
      (1) Minor operation—1.2
      (2) Skeletal trauma—1.35
      (3) Major sepsis—1.6
      (4) Severe thermal burn—2.10

[†]BEE = basal energy expenditure; W = weight (kg); H = height (cm); and A = age.

Harris–Benedict Equation and Calvin Long—Activity Factor reprinted with permission from Berk, J., and Sampliner, J. Handbook of Critical Care, 3rd ed. Boston: Little, Brown, 1990.

chapter 6

BLOOD, BLOOD COMPONENTS, AND VOLUME EXPANDERS

BLOOD TRANSFUSIONS

USE OF ALTERNATIVE BLOOD GROUPS

In critical emergency situations, when blood of ABO compatibility is not available, an alternative ABO group may be used. When making the decision to use blood of an alternative group, risks and benefits to the *individual* patient should be carefully considered. However, when units of an ABO group *other* than the patient's have been transfused, subsequent units should be transfused *only* after a posttransfusion crossmatch is obtained for the possibility of anti-A or anti-B in the recipient's serum. The decision to revert to the patient's *own* type should be based on compatibility testing and serum groupings carried through to the antiglobulin test.

Whole Blood and Red Blood Cells

Patient's ABO Group	1st Choice	2nd Choice	3rd Choice
O Positive	O Positive (WB or PRBC)[†]	O Negative (WB or PRBC)	
O Negative	O Negative (WB or PRBC)		O Positive in *extreme* emergency
A Positive	A Positive (WB or PRBC)	O Positive (PRBC)	A or O Negative (PRBC)
A Negative	A Negative (WB or PRBC)	O Negative (PRBC)	A or O Negative (PRBC)
B Positive	B Positive (WB or PRBC)	O Positive (PRBC)	B or O Negative (PRBC)
B Negative	B Negative (WB or PRBC)	O Negative (PRBC)	O or B Positive in *extreme* emergency (PRBC only)
AB Positive	AB Positive (WB or PRBC)	A Positive (PRBC) or B Positive (PRBC)	O Positive (PRBC) Any negative PRBC in *extreme* emergency
AB Negative	AB Negative (WB or PRBC)	A Negative (PRBC) or B Negative (PRBC)	O Negative (PRBC) A Positive PRBC in *extreme* emergency

---

[†]WB = whole blood; PRBC = packed red blood cells.

Fresh Frozen Plasma‡

Patient's ABO Group	*1st Choice*	*2nd Choice*
O Positive	O Positive	O Negative
O Negative	O Negative	
A Positive	A Positive	A Negative
A Negative	A Negative	
B Positive	B Positive	B Negative
B Negative	B Negative or B Positive	AB Negative or AB Positive
AB Positive	AB Positive	AB Negative
AB Negative	AB Negative	

Platelets

Patient's ABO Group	*Selection*
Group O	Any group platelets may be administered
Group A	If available, A or AB platelets should be administered
Group B	B platelets are preferable, but any group available can be administered

---

‡The donor plasma and the recipient RBCs should be ABO compatible.

BLOOD TRANSFUSION REACTION CHART

In the event of suspected reaction, the transfusion should be discontinued *immediately* and the vein kept open with an appropriate solution.

Reaction	Etiology	Signs/Symptoms	Intervention	Prevention
Hemolytic (Uncommon, possibly fatal)	• ABO or Rh incompatibility • Improper storage of blood	• Anxiety • Tachycardia/ tachypnea • Chills • Fever • Low back pain • Chest pain • Hypotension • Nausea • Vomiting • Bleeding abnormalities	• Initiate emergency measures (O_2, fluids, emergency drugs) • Maintain renal function • Collect blood, urine samples	• Minimize risk by – validation of patient/unit compatibility per hospital policy • Begin transfusion slowly • Monitor vital signs per hospital policy
Allergic (Common, serious)	• Atopic substance in the blood • Previous sensitization or congenital IgA deficiency	• Pruritis, urticaria • Chills • Vomiting, cramping • Severe diarrhea • Severe dyspnea, wheezing • Hypotension	• Same as above • Antihistamine, epinephrine or steroids as ordered	• Minimize risk by – knowledge of patient history of previous allergic transfusion reaction, if any

Febrile (Most common transfusion reaction)	• Bacterial, lipopolysaccharides in blood
	• Pregnancy
	• Transfusion of 5 or more units of blood (recipient antibody screening should be done after multiple transfusions)
		• Chills/fever
		• Tachycardia
		• Palpitations
		• Flushing
		• Muscle aches (may resemble hemolytic reaction)
			• Antipyretics
			• Antihistamine as ordered
				• Minimize risk by
				  – keeping the patient covered and warm
				  – using saline washed cells or frozen saline washed packed cells
				  – giving antipyretics with the blood

Bacterial (Uncommon, serious)	• Presence of endotoxins in blood
	• Immunosuppressed patients are at high risk
		• Severe abdominal cramping
		• Sudden hyperthermia
		• Abrupt vomiting
		• Shaking chills
		• Hypotension
			• Antibiotics and steroids as ordered	• Minimize risk by
				  – adhering to strict aseptic technique in handling blood and transfusion equipment
				  – changing tubing and filter after every unit
				  – not allowing blood to hang more than 4 hr

BLOOD TRANSFUSION REACTION CHART *Continued*

Reaction	Etiology	Signs/Symptoms	Intervention	Prevention

Circulatory Overload (Common, treatable)	• Excessive volume
	• Rapid infusion
	• Fluid shift from administration of albumin
		• Dry cough (initially)
		• Chest tightness
		• Restlessness
		• Dyspnea
		• Basilar rales on auscultation
		• Jugular venous distention
		• Eventually acute pulmonary edema
			• Keep vein open with D_5W (not saline solution)
			• Diuretics
			• Rotating tourniquets per order
				• Minimize risk by
				  – using packed cells
				  – reducing infusion rate for susceptible patients
				  – per order, using diuretic at beginning of transfusion

Air Embolism (Uncommon, possibly fatal)	• Air introduced via infusion tubing	• Shortness of breath
		• Chest pain
		• Cough
		• Hypotension
		• Possible cardiac arrest
			• Treat for shock
			• Turn patient to left side, head down
				• Minimize risk by
				  – purging tubing prior to beginning infusion
				  – maintaining seal at connector sites
				  – not allowing blood bag to run dry

PRODUCTS

All blood and blood components must be verified according to hospital policy.

WHOLE BLOOD

Description

Complete
unadulterated
blood

Indications

- Anemia
- Severe blood loss
- Hypovolemia

Contraindications

- When volume increase would be detrimental
- Availability of specific, needed components

Administration Technique

- Administration by straight-line, Y, or microaggregate set
- Large bore needle or catheter (18–19 ga)
- Change administration set with each unit

Nursing/Medical Implications

- Crossmatch necessary
- ABO and Rh must be *exact* match
- Rate: 2–4 hr/unit
- Do not obtain blood until ready for transfusion (cannot be returned to the blood bank)
- Monitor closely during transfusion for signs of transfusion reaction (see transfusion reaction chart, pp. 222–224)

RED BLOOD CELLS (PACKED OR FROZEN)

Description	Indications	Contraindications	Administration Technique	Nursing/Medical Implications
Whole blood with 80% of the supernatant plasma removed	• Correction of RBC loss – hemolysis, sickle cell anemia, drug poisoning, thalas-semia, bone marrow depression, chronic renal failure • Prevention of circulatory overload in congested states	• Anemia related to hematopoietic nutrients; iron, vitamin B-12, folic acid	• Same as whole blood	• Same as whole blood

WASHED RED BLOOD CELLS

Description	Indications	Contraindications	Administration Technique	Nursing/Medical Implications
RBCs with 20% plasma	• Documented plasma protein antibodies or transfusion reaction to WBCs • Transfusion therapy when WBC antibody stimulation is undesirable		• Regular blood administration set (microaggregates removed during washing) • Administer immediately. Cells expire 24 hr after washing	• Same as whole blood

WHITE BLOOD CELLS

Description
Whole blood with all the RBCs and 80% of the supernatant plasma removed

Indications
- Life threatening granulocytopenia (radiation induced)
- Predisposition to infection resulting from immunosuppression

Contraindications
- Granulocyte transfusions contraindicated in *absence* of profound granulocytopenia (<100 cells/uL)
- Transfusions may be withheld when bone marrow recovery expected

Administration Technique
- Microaggregate filter *should not* be used
- Rate: 2–4 hr/unit

Nursing/Medical Implications
- Crossmatch necessary
- ABO compatible; HLA preferred
- Pheresis *cannot* remove every RBC; allergic reaction and hemolysis *may occur*
- Fever and shaking chills may be *desired* response as circulating granulocytes begin phagocytosis
- Stop transfusion if graft vs. host reaction occurs in immunosuppressed patient
- Recipient should be protected from sources of potential infection

PLASMA (FRESH OR FRESH FROZEN)

Description	Indications	Contraindications	Administration Technique	Nursing/Medical Implications
Uncoagulated plasma separated from whole blood	• Clotting factor deficiency when specific concentrate is not available • Hypovolemia • Hepatic disease • Prevention dilutional hypocoagulability and hypoproteinemia	• When specific therapy for coagulation anomaly is available or when albumin only is necessary	• Administer by any straight-line set • Normal saline not necessary for Y-set; concentrate contains no RBCs • Plasma used to replace coagulation factors should be administered through filter • Microaggregate (40–20 μ) are *contraindicated* as they trap plasma • Smaller needles may be used (21–23 ga) • Expires 24 hr after thawing	• Crossmatch not necessary • Need not be ABO identical but should be RBC compatible • Can be given regardless of Rh type • Administer as rapidly as possible, depending on patient • Monitor for allergic urticaria or elevated temperature • Plasma may appear cloudy, greenish, or yellow, depending on donor's diet or estrogen intake

PLATELETS

Description

Platelet sediment from platelet-rich plasma resuspended in 30–50 mL of plasma

Indications

- Decreased platelet production from leukemia or bone marrow suppression
- Platelet destruction from drugs or immune system disorders
- Dilutional thrombocytopenia resulting from massive blood transfusions
- Vitamin B-12 or folic acid deficiency

Contraindications

- Bleeding unrelated to abnormal platelet function or decreased platelet concentration
- Post transfusion purpura or thrombotic thrombocytopenia

Administration Technique

- Special platelet filter
- Do not use standard blood filter

Nursing/Medical Implications

- Crossmatch not necessary
- ABO compatibility
- Administer as rapidly as possible, uninterrupted
- Two units per kg/ body weight raises platelet count by 50,000/cu mm
- Administer antihistamine before transfusion to patients with history of side effects

PLASMA PROTEIN FRACTION (PPF)

Description
5% solution of selected protein from pooled plasma in buffered stabilized saline diluent

Indications
- Volume expansion
- Hypovolemic shock
- Hypoproteinemia

Contraindications
- In clotting factory deficiency; all coagulation factors are absent from PPF

Administration Technique
- Straight-line set

Nursing/Medical Implications
- Crossmatch not necessary
- Infuse at rate and volume consistent with patient response
- PPF contains ≥85% albumin
- Observe for signs of pulmonary edema, fluid overload
- Monitor for sudden hypotension
- Monitor serum sodium level
- Use cautiously in presence of renal or hepatic failure

ALBUMIN 5% (BUFFERED SALINE) AND ALBUMIN 25% (SALT POOR)

Description

Heat treated, aqueous, chemically processed fraction of pooled plasma

Indications

- Hypoproteinemia
- Shock states (burns, trauma, infection, surgery)
- Maintenance of electrolyte balance
- Prevention of hemoconcentration

Contraindications

- Severe anemia
- Cardiac failure

Administration Technique

- Administer per provided set

Nursing/Medical Implications

- Crossmatch not necessary
- Administer rapidly to patient in shock
- Administer slowly (1 mg/min) to patient with hyperproteinemia or with adequate blood volume
- May be diluted with saline or 5% dextrose in water
- May be substituted for whole blood as volume expander while crossmatch is being accomplished
- Sterilized by pasteurization; carries minimal risk of transmitting hepatitis

CRYOPRECIPITATE

Description	Indications	Contraindications	Administration Technique	Nursing/Medical Implications
Cold insoluble portion of plasma recovered from fresh frozen plasma	• Altered clotting profile associated with decreased levels of Factor VIII *and* fibrogen		• Administer by syringe or component drip set *only* • Gauge needle: 22 or 23 • Rate: 1 U/5 min (as rapidly as possible) • Flush line with saline to ensure complete transfusion of cryoprecipitate • Administer as soon as possible after thawing to reduce loss of activity	• Crossmatch unnecessary (donor) plasma and recipient RBC should be ABO compatible) • Initial dose: 1 U/6 kg of body weight; subsequent doses: 1 U/12 kg of body weight at 6–8 hr intervals • Possible adverse effects include urticaria, chills, tremors • Hepatitis risk same as with whole blood

ANTIHEMOPHILIC FACTOR (AHF, AHG, AND FACTOR VIII)

Description

A lyophilized powder prepared by cold precipitation from pooled plasma

Indications

- Prevention/control of bleeding in patients with factor VIII deficiency
- Hemophilia A
- Acquired factor VIII deficiency

Contraindications

- Not effective for treating von Willebrand's disease

Administration Technique

- Administer with filter needle provided with product
- Plastic syringe only should be used; AHF solution adheres to glass syringes
- Freeze dried; reconstitute with diluent provided
- Diluent and powder should be at room temperature prior to reconstitution; use within 3 hr
- Rate: as rapidly as patient can tolerate to a maximum of 6 mL/min

Nursing/Medical Implications

- Monitor pulse rate while infusing
- Reactions include headache, somnolence, loss of consciousness, tachycardia, hypotension, fever, chills, urticaria, nausea, vomiting
- Most side effects subside within 15–20 min and may be rate related
- Hepatitis risk same as with whole blood

**Concentrations of AHF may vary with specific brands.
Read manufacturer's literature prior to administration.**

FACTOR IX COMPLEX

Description

Lyophilized concentrate of coagulation factors II, VII, IX, and X derived from fresh plasma

Indications

- Hemophilia B (Christmas disease)
- Factor IX deficiency

Contraindications

- Used for factor IX deficiency only

Administration Technique

- Administer with filter needle provided with product
- Freeze dried; reconstitute with diluent provided
- May be administered by direct IV push or IV infusion
- Diluent and powder should be at room temperature prior to reconstitution. Use within 3 hr
- Rate: 100 U/min usually well tolerated; do not exceed 10 mL/min

Nursing/Medical Implications

- Transient fever, chills, headache, tingling, flushing, changes in B/P and pulse
- DIC reported in patients receiving factor IX; monitor coagulation studies
- Risk of hepatitis same as with whole blood

DEXTRAN 40, 70, AND 75

Description
Blood volume expander

Indications
- Shock: dextran increases plasma volume and improves circulation
- Prophylaxis of venous thrombosis or pulmonary emboli in surgery that has high risk of embolic complications

Contraindications
- Thrombocytopenia
- Clotting disorders
- Impaired renal function
- Pulmonary edema
- CHF
- Dehydration (dextran 40)

Administration Technique
- Use only clear solutions
- Discard unused portions
- If blood is to be administered, change tubing and flush well between dextran and blood; dextran causes slight coagulation in tubing

Nursing/Medical Implications
- Therapy should not continue for more than 5 days
- Heparin given with dextran 70 or 75 may profoundly depress clotting capabilities
- Blood glucose determinations may yield false high values
- Crossmatching may not be accurate because of interference from dextran
- Observe for cardiovascular overload, edema
- Hematocrit may be reduced but should not be allowed to fall below 30%

DEXTRAN 40, 70, AND 75   *Continued*

- Side effects may include nausea, vomiting, stool incontinence, urticaria, wheezing, chest tightness, hypotension
- Hydration should be kept adequate to maintain urine flow
- Mark lab requisitions "Dextran"

HETASTARCH 6% IN 0.9% NACL

Description	Indications	Contraindications	Administration Technique	Nursing/Medical Implications
Blood substitute	• Increases plasma volume • Shock • Adjunct in leukapheresis to improve harvesting and yield of granulocytes	• Severe bleeding disorders • CHF • Renal failure	• IV administration only • Use only clear solutions • Discard unused portions • Rate: variable, depending on patient response • Reduce rate for burns or septic shock • Change IV tubing or flush with saline before giving blood	• Can interfere with platelet function • Side effects may include increased arterial and venous pressure, increased stroke volume and cardiac workload, fever, chills, itching, vomiting, headache, anaphylaxis

AUTOLOGOUS TRANSFUSION

Autotransfusion is the reclamation and reuse of patients' own blood. Shed blood may be salvaged from body cavities, joint spaces, and other operative or trauma sites. The use of autologous blood avoids problems of incompatibility and transmission of disease and is economically feasible. Patients who object to homologous transfusion *may* consent to the use of autologous blood.

Advantages
- Safer than homologous blood; avoids
  - allergic reaction
  - incompatibility
  - blood borne disease
- Viable red blood cells
- Rapid availability
- *May be* acceptable to patients who object to homologous tranfusion
- Cost effective

Indications
- Rare blood types
- Multiple known antibodies
- Prior transfusion complications
- Surgery
  - intraoperative salvage
  - total hip/knee replacement
  - spinal fusions
  - coronary artery bypass graft
  - vascular surgery/ruptured aortic aneurysm
  - surgeries involving liver and spleen
  - ectopic pregnancy

Indications   *Continued*
 – thoracic surgery
 – neurosurgery
 – urologic surgery
 – major plastic/reconstructive surgery
- Emergency
 – trauma
 – hemothorax
 – injuries involving liver, spleen

Contraindications
- Wound contamination with urine or feces
- Bacteremia
- Malignancy
- Cesarean section; potential for amniotic fluid emboli
- Blood dyscrasia, coagulopathies

Complications
- Sepsis secondary to contamination
- Microembolism
- Hemolysis
- Coagulopathy (DIC)

Process
- Preoperative donation
 – controlled phlebotomy of a cannulated vein
 – may be collected 500 cc weekly until desired amount obtained
 – last donation should *not* be within 72 hr of anticipated use
 – blood to be stored must be anticoagulated

- Perioperative donation
  - controlled phlebotomy of a cannulated vein
  - collected just prior to use
  - should be replaced with equal amount of crystalline or colloidal solution
    - crystalline replacement includes Lactated Ringer's, infused at three times amount of blood withdrawn
    - colloidal replacement includes hetastarch, pentastarch, dextran, and human albumin
  - hemodilution contraindicated in patients suffering anemia or renal failure, cardiac dysfunction, severe hepatic disease, COPD
- Intraoperative salvage
  - blood salvaged from operative site or extracorporeal circuit may require "washing" to remove nonblood components, such as povidone–iodine
  - blood salvaged from orthopedic procedure does *not* demonstrate defibrination and requires anticoagulation
- Postoperative salvage
  - shed blood salvaged from body cavities, joint spaces, and other closed operative or trauma sites
    - hip or knee replacement
    - thoracic surgery
    - noncontaminated wounds

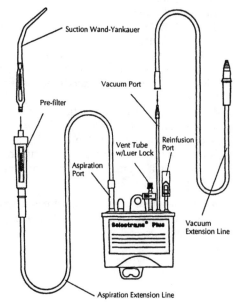

Figure 6.1 Solcotrans® Plus Intraoperative Autotransfusion System

Solcotrans® is a registered trademark of C.R. Bard, Inc. Reprinted with permission from Davol Inc. (P.O. Box 8500, Cranston, RI 02920), 1995.

– may require special processing (washing) to remove debris and contaminates (i.e., free hemoglobin, cellular debris, fibrin, bone particles, activated clotting factors, platelets)

– adverse effects of unwashed blood include DIC, renal failure, ARDS, emboli consisting of fatty particles, activated clotting factors, other debris

• Trauma

– blood salvaged from traumatic wounds

– contraindications include

– grossly contaminated blood

– blood from a wound more than 4 hr old

– patients with compromised renal or hepatic function

Reinfusion of autologous blood must begin within 6 hr of *starting* collection. NOT INTENDED FOR STORAGE.

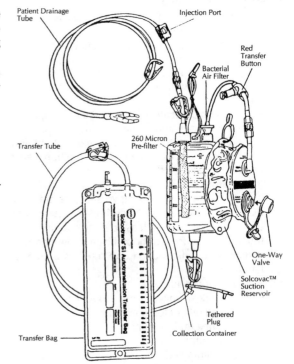

Figure 6.2 Solcotrans® SI Orthopaedic Autotransfusion System

Reprinted with permission from Davol Inc., 1995.

chapter 7

EQUIPMENT

GASTROINTESTINAL INTUBATION

UPPER GI DISORDERS

The physician will choose a tube appropriate to the patient's need. Introduction and maintenance of any tube should comply with institutional requirements, policies, and protocol. The tube should not interfere with the patient's breathing. Before instilling anything in a tube verify its placement. Monitor the patient for dehydration and electrolyte imbalance. The head of the bed should be elevated to 45° before introducing tube feedings or medications.

Tube	Description	Indications	Nursing/Medical Implications
Salem Sump 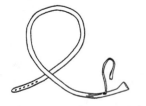 **Figure 7.1** Salem Sump Tube	• Double lumen • 48 in. (122 cm) – marked at 45, 55, 65, and 75 cm • Clear plastic with radiopaque line • Blue sump port (pigtail) allows introduction of atmospheric air to patient's stomach; prevents tube from adhering to and damaging gastric mucosa • Larger lumen serves as suction tube	• Aspiration of gastric fluids and gases • Gastric lavage • Diagnostic studies • Enteral feeding • Drug administration	• Blue pigtail should be kept above level of patient's stomach to prevent gastric reflux • Irrigate large lumen as necessary *then* introduce air into pigtail lumen

Levin

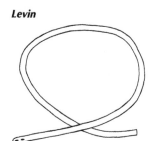

Figure 7.2   Levin Tube

- Single lumen
- 42–50 in. (107–127 cm)
  – marked at 45, 55, 65, and 75 cm
- Rubber or plastic
- Holes along side and at tip

- Aspiration of gastric fluids and gases
- Gastric lavage
- Diagnostic studies
- Enteral feeding
- Drug administration

- When 2nd marker of tube is entering nares (about 55 cm), tube should be in stomach

Ewald

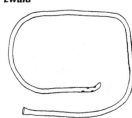

Figure 7.3   Ewald Tube

- Single lumen
- Large bore
- Several openings at distal end
- Allows use of large volume of irrigants to enter and leave stomach rapidly

- Gastric lavage
  – bleeding
  – drug overdose
  – ingestion of poison

- For short-term use; should be removed after lavage and evacuation of gastric content

Tube	Description	Indications	Nursing/Medical Implications
Moss 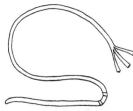 **Figure 7.4** Moss Tube	• Triple lumen • 20 Fr. tube • First lumen (balloon inflation port) positioned and inflated at cardia • Second lumen serves as esophagogastric aspiration tube • Third lumen is duodenal feeding port • Radiopaque tip	• Prevention of post-operative ileus • Aspiration of stomach contents after surgery • Duodenal feeding postoperatively	• Tube placed intraoperatively
Levacuator 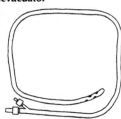 **Figure 7.5** Levacuator Tube	• Double lumen • Large bore • Large lumen allows evacuation of gastric contents • Small lumen is for instillation of irrigant	• Gastric lavage – bleeding – drug overdose – ingestion of poison	• Short-term use • Remove after lavage and evacuation of gastric contents

Edlich

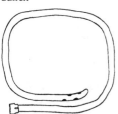

Figure 7.6 Edlich Tube

- Single lumen
- Large bore
- Distal tip closed
- Four openings in distal lumen

- Gastric lavage
  - bleeding
  - poison ingestion
  - drug overdose

- Short-term use
- Remove after lavage and evacuation of gastric contents

Duo-Feed

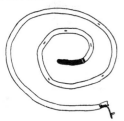

Figure 7.7 Duo-Feed Tube

- Small bore
- Extremely flexible
- 102 cm
- Outer PVC tube
- Inner silicone catheter

- Enteral feeding

- Reduces discomfort, reflux, esophageal erosion, fistula formulation
- Requires stylet to facilitate insertion
- X-ray chest before initiating tube feedings

LOWER GI DISORDERS

Tube	Description	Indications	Nursing/Medical Implications

Cantor
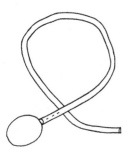
Figure 7.8 Cantor Tube
	• Single lumen
	• 10 ft. (3 m)
	• 16 Fr.
	• Balloon at distal end for mercury instillation
		• Aspiration of bowel contents
		• Relief of bowel obstruction
			• Prior to insertion
			  – fill balloon bag's upper chamber with mercury
			  – aspirate all air from bag
			
			Mercury must be handled in compliance with institutional requirements.

Harris
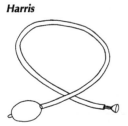
Figure 7.9 Harris Tube
	• Single lumen
	• 6 ft. (1.8 m)
	• Metal tip
	• Balloon for mercury instillation
		• Aspiration of bowel contents
		• Relief of bowel obstruction
		• Lavage of intestinal tract
			• Prior to insertion
			  – fill balloon bag's upper chamber with mercury
			  – aspirate all air from bag
			
			Mercury must be handled in compliance with institutional requirements.

Miller–Abbott

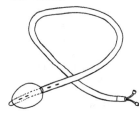

Figure 7.10 Miller–Abbott Tube

- Double lumen
  - one lumen for balloon inflation
  - one lumen for drainage or suction
- 10 ft. (3 m)
- Ranges in size from 12– 18 Fr.

- Aspiration of bowel contents
- Relief of bowel obstruction
- Dilatation of bowel

- Label each lumen
- Fill balloon with mercury when tube reaches the stomach
- Clamp balloon lumen; prevents accidental loss of mercury through suctioning

Mercury must be handled in compliance with institutional requirements.

ESOPHAGEAL TUBES

The physician inserts esophageal tubes. They are designed to control or stop esophageal bleeding but may also precipitate complications such as airway obstruction, esophageal edema, ulceration, or necrosis.

Tube	Description	Indications	Nursing/Medical Implications
Minnesota	• Four-lumen tube – gastric balloon inflation lumen with gastric balloon pressure monitoring port **Gastric balloon inflation capacity is 450–500 cc.**	• Stop or control esophageal bleeding	• Make sure each lumen is clearly identified • Esophageal balloon should not be inflated for more than 24 hr • Gastric balloon should be inflated for 24 hr after bleeding ceases

Esophageal aspiration lumen
Gastric aspiration lumen
Gastric balloon--inflation lumen
Gastric balloon
pressure--monitoring port

Esophageal balloon
pressure--monitoring port

Esophageal balloon--inflation lumen

Esophageal balloon
Gastric balloon

Figure 7.11 Minnesota Tube

Tube	Description	Indications	Nursing/Medical Implications
	– esophageal balloon inflation lumen with esophageal pressure monitoring port – gastric aspiration lumen – esophageal aspiration lumen		• Gastric balloon should be deflated, traction released and left in place for 24–36 hr or until gastric aspirate is clear
Sengstaken–Blakemore 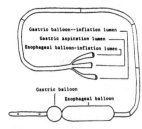 **Figure 7.12** Sengstaken–Blakemore Tube	• Triple lumen – gastric balloon inflation lumen **Gastric balloon capacity is 200–250 cc.** – esophageal balloon inflation lumen **Esophageal balloon inflation capacity is 30–45 mm Hg.** – gastric aspiration lumen	• Control of esophageal bleeding	• Esophageal balloon should be maintained at lowest pressure that will control bleeding • Esophageal balloon should be deflated 12–24 hr prior to withdrawal • If bleeding recurs, balloon pressure should be reestablished immediately • Patient cannot swallow saliva and may require a nasogastric tube to aspirate secretions that collect about esophageal balloon

In the figure:
Gastric balloon--inflation lumen
Gastric aspiration lumen
Esophageal balloon-inflation lumen
Gastric balloon
Esophageal balloon

Linton–Nachlas

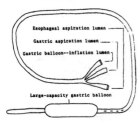

Esophageal aspiration lumen
Gastric aspiration lumen
Gastric balloon--inflation lumen

Large-capacity gastric balloon

Figure 7.13 Linton–Nachlas Tube

- Triple lumen
  – gastric balloon inflation lumen

Balloon capacity is 700–800 cc.
  – gastric aspiration lumen
  – esophageal aspiration lumen

- Control of esophageal bleeding

- Use of tube for longer than 40 hr may cause cardioesophageal junction necrosis

WOUND DRAIN DEVICES

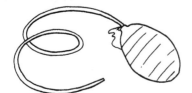

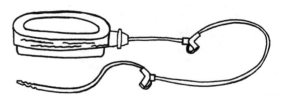

Figure 7.14A   Jackson–Pratt Drain Device   **Figure 7.14B**   Hemovac Drain Device

Functions
- To withdraw accumulated fluid/secretions from a wound or surgical site
- To facilitate healing from inside out

Indications
- Large amounts of drainage
- Drainage that may prevent healing
- Closed wound drainage

Advantages
- Antireflux valve prevents backflow
- Gentle suction prevents tissue damage
- May be used with wall suction
- Does not limit patient mobility

Nursing/Medical Implications
- Drains are available in an array of configurations and capabilities
- Generally removed 3–7 days postoperatively but may remain longer if necessary
- Silicone coated and with numerous perforations; occlusions are rare
- System may be irrigated if occlusion suspected
- Maintain sterile technique

URINARY DIVERSION DEVICES

Diversion of urine may be necessary as a result of genitourinary disease, trauma, or surgery. Management should comply with institutional policies and procedures.

Device	**Description**	**Indications**	**Nursing/Medical Implications**
Nephrostomy Tube 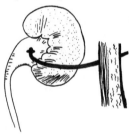 **Figure 7.15** Nephrostomy Tube	• Teflon-coated latex catheter • Balloon tipped	• Drainage of urine directly from kidney – urinary tract obstruction – cystectomy – neurogenic bladder – prostatic cancer – congenital defects • Trauma to renal tissue • Permanent loss of ureteral function	• Hematuria expected for 24–48 hr after placement • Tube should be checked frequently for obstruction; nephrostomy tube should never be clamped • Obstructed tube may cause kidney damage; renal pelvis holds only 5–8 cc • Maintain closed drainage system

Device
Ureteral Stent

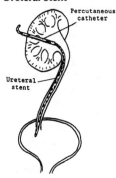

Figure 7.16   Ureteral Stent

Description
- Radiopaque dacron and nylon or polyurethane catheter
- Available in numerous configurations, depending on specific need

Indications
- Maintenance of urinary flow in patients with ureteral obstruction
- Maintenance of ureter size and patency after surgery

Nursing/Medical Implications
- May be used along with indwelling foley catheter
- Tube may be irrigated (per physician order) *to maintain patency,* but never to lavage the kidney
- Ureteral stent is placed via cystoscopy
- Stent dislodgement may cause colicky pain and decreased urinary output

IMPLANTABLE INFUSION DEVICES: CENTRAL VENOUS CATHETERS

Venous access devices, generally referred to as central venous catheters (CVC), are used to administer fluids, blood, blood products, or TPN and to obtain blood specimens. Arterial, peritoneal, and intrathecal access is used for administering drugs regionally *only*.

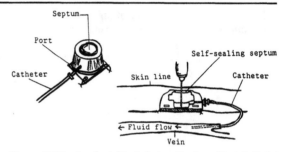

Figure 7.17 Implantable Infusion Devices (Port-A-Cath/Infuse-A-Port)

Device	Description	Indications	Nursing/Medical Implications
Port-A-Cath	• Polyurethane or silicone catheter • Plastic, stainless steel, or titanium port • Thick rubber septum covers port reservoir • Available in single or double lumen	• Prolonged drug and fluid administration • Blood administration • Chemotherapy • TPN • Lab sampling	• No external parts • Implanted for long-term use in a subcutaneous pocket in chest wall • Cannula positioned in internal jugular or subclavian vein **Arterial access may be used for regional drug delivery and should be used for that specific therapy only. Arterial cannulation is not acceptable for routine medications, IVs, or lab sampling.** • Access port cannulated via Huber needle; for continuous infusion, Huber needle may be secured in place and left for several days; for intermittent infusion, needle may be left in port and system heparinized after each use

Infuse-A-Port

- Radiopaque silicone rubber catheter
- Access port contains self-sealing septum
- Flange with holes for suturing device in place

- Repeated or prolonged access to vascular system
  - blood sampling
  - injection
  - infusion therapy
  - delivery of imaging solutions

- Implanted in subcutaneous pocket of chest wall
- Meant for long-term use

Arterial access may be used for regional drug delivery and should be used for that specific therapy only. Arterial cannulation is not acceptable for routine medications, IVs, or lab sampling.

- Intraperitoneal access may be used for regional chemotherapy
- Port is cannulated by using a special Infusaid needle
- System should be heparinized to prevent clotting and loss of device

Device	Description	Indications	Nursing/Medical Implications
Broviac/Hickman Catheter 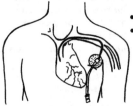 **Figure 7.18** Broviac/ Hickman Catheter	• Silicone rubber catheter (more biocompatible than polyurethane) • Radiopaque • Single or double lumen	• Long-term venous access • Continuous or intermittent IV therapy • Chemotherapy • TPN • Lab sampling • Blood or blood products transfusion	• Placement is surgical procedure, using fluoroscopy • Injection cap located externally on chest wall • Catheter is threaded into circulatory system via venous cutdown or percutaneous access • Cephalic vein most commonly used but external jugular is acceptable • Catheter stabilized by growth of subcutaneous tissue over a dacron cuff located 30 cm from hub; growth takes place in about 10–14 days • Catheter available for use immediately

- As with all such devices, care must be taken to prevent opening system and allowing either air embolization or bleeding
- Large bore lumen of Hickman precludes occlusion
- Broviac lumen is smaller; preferred for children and patient with veins of poor integrity
- Catheter fractures may be repaired by using a 14-ga, 2-in. angiocath or by using commercially available repair kit
- Requires heparinization
- Patient activity is, essentially, unrestricted after subcutaneous overgrowth takes place and patient is able to care for device

Device
Groshong

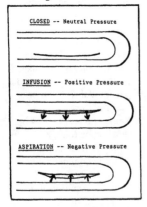

Figure 7.19 Groshong Catheter Tip

Description

- Soft silastic catheter
- Obturator wire used for catheter insertion
- Radiopaque
- Replaceable leur-lock injection cap
- Closed tip with three-way, pressure-sensitive valve
- Single or multiple lumen
- Dacron cuff promotes stability through fibrin growth and prevents migration of organisms up catheter lumen

Indications

- Long-term venous access
- Parenteral nutrition
- Lab sampling
- Medication delivery (i.e., chemotherapy)

Nursing/Medical Implications

- Access sites of choice: internal or external jugular vein
- Does not require heparinization
- Flush with normal saline
  – should be "brisk" to ensure that blood or other substances have cleared valve before closure
- No clamping required
- Repair of proximal end of catheter easily accomplished; using repair kit available from manufacturer
  – clean catheter end with povidone iodine
  – cut damaged end off catheter (use sterile scissors)
  – detach protector sleeve from connector hub

- slide sleeve onto catheter
- insert replacement connector hub into catheter by using provided stylet for support
- push connector shaft into catheter until end of catheter firmly seated against base of hub
- discard stylet; flush catheter with 20 cc of normal saline
- Groshong insertion is reverse of other vascular access devices: tunneled *from* venous access site *to* exit site
- Potential for air embolism or accidental blood loss reduced
- Complications include: site infection, sepsis, venous thrombosis, broken hub cap
- Occluded catheter may be cleared with urokinase

Device	Description	Indications	Nursing/Medical Implications
Peripherally Inserted Central Catheter (PICC) 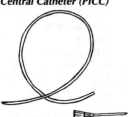 **Figure 7.20** Peripherally Inserted Central Venous Catheter	• Silicone rubber catheter	• Short-term home therapy (2–6 weeks) • Chest injury precluding use of device that has exit site on chest wall • Patients at risk of infection from breaching skin on chest wall • Patient who already has CVC on chest • Therapy of such short duration that patients choose not to undergo surgical procedure for placement	• Peripherally inserted through standard peripheral catheter • Veins of choice are cephalic or basilic • Exit port is placed in anticubital space • Patient mobility of involved extremity is limited • Reduced risk for thrombus formation • Catheter repair easily accomplished by using repair kit

MONITORING SYSTEMS

INTRACRANIAL PRESSURE MONITORING

Normal Valves

- Intracranial pressure normally ranges from 110–140 mm H_2O or 0–10 mm Hg
- Cerebral blood flow (CBF) = mean arterial pressure (MAP) – intracranial pressure (ICP)
- Cerebral perfusion pressure (CPP) = MAP (approximately)
    - normal CPP is 80–90 mm Hg; minimum of 50 mm Hg necessary to perfuse the brain; below that, ischemia and death can result
    - cerebral blood flow ceases when ICP equals CPP

Indications
- Neoplasm
- Cerebral edema
- Intracranial hemorrhage
- Cerebral aneurysm
- Near drowning
- Hydrocephalus
- Encephalitis

Monitoring Techniques
Intraventricular Catheter
- Advantages
  - provides the most reliable waveforms
  - permits drainage of cerebrospinal fluid (CSF) from a lateral ventricle to decrease pressure
  - allows pressure response testing; measuring compliance of cranial compartment
  - affords access to CSF pathway
  - provides route for intraventricular medications/ contrast media
- Disadvantages
  - catheter may be difficult to place, especially if ventricle has been distorted by increased intracranial pressure (ICP)
  - catheter may damage cerebral tissue during placement
  - increases risk of infection
  - may cause excessive CSF drainage resulting in life-threatening drop in ICP
  - difficult to maintain patency of the catheter
  - severely restricts patient's mobility

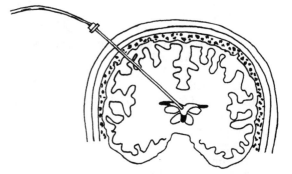

Figure 7.21   Intraventricular Catheter

- Procedure
  - intraventricular catheter placed in anterior horn of lateral ventricle through drill hole in skull
  - placement usually in nondominant hemisphere
- Nursing/Medical Implications
  - catheter patency should be monitored frequently
  - if irrigation required, must be accomplished by physician
  - stopcock must be properly positioned; improper positioning may allow excessive drainage of CSF, resulting in precipitous drop in ICP and formation of subdural hematoma
  - sudden changes in ICP reading may indicate compressed catheter giving false reading as a result of collapsed ventricles
  - transducer and monitor should be recalibrated frequently; transducer level should be approximately at ear canal level

Subarachnoid Screw
- Advantages
  - less invasive
  - insertion quicker and less risky
  - patient has more mobility
  - potential for infection diminished
  - allows accurate ICP readings for patients whose ventricles are too small to accommodate intraventricular catheter
  - *small amounts* of CSF can be drained to decrease ICP or obtain lab specimens
- Disadvantages
  - risk of brain herniation
  - risk of CSF leakage
  - increased potential for infection
  - may not be used to drain significant amounts of CSF

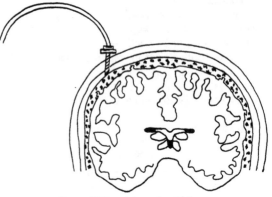

Figure 7.22 Subarachnoid Screw

- screw may be occluded by blood or brain tissue
- contrast media cannot be instilled
- contraindicated in children under 5 because of instability of cranial bones
- Procedure
  - steel screw with sensor tip is inserted through drill burr hole in skull; small incision is made in dura mater allowing screw and tip to enter subarachnoid space; transducer attached to screw converts CSF pressure to electrical impulse
- Nursing/Medical Implications
  - frequent monitoring of screw patency is imperative
  - if the screw becomes occluded, *physician* may irrigate it
  - recalibrate transducer and monitor frequently
  - monitor closely for signs of infection

Epidural Probe
- Advantages
  - least invasive method if ICP monitoring; dura is not penetrated
  - lowest infection risk
  - easiest, quickest insertion
  - optimal patient mobility
- Disadvantages
  - epidural reading may not be consistent with intraventricular pressure as sensor is placed outside dura
  - intracranial compliance cannot be tested
  - CSF specimens cannot be obtained
  - some types of epidural probes cannot be recalibrated; newer models connect to a pressure module that can be recalibrated

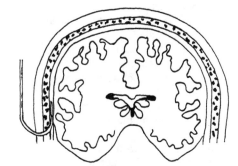

Figure 7.23 Epidural Probe

- Procedure
  - a fiberoptic sensor is placed between the skull and the dura (epidural space) through a burr hole
- Nursing/Medical Implications
  - monitor the patency of pressure module connections
  - observe closely for signs of infection

Intraparenchymal Monitoring System

- Advantages
  - selectively measures ICP in brain parenchyma
  - decreased risk of infection
  - ease of placement
- Disadvantages
  - requires separate monitoring systems
  - unable to drain CSF
  - fracture of fiberoptic cable
  - cannot be recalibrated
  - sensor may cause tissue damage
- Procedure
  - a small fiberoptic transducer tipped sensor is placed directly into the brain tissue just below the subarachnoid space
  - the fiberoptic probe is connected via its fiberoptic cable to a bedside monitor
- Nursing/Medical Implications
  - maintain ICP monitoring device to ensure accuracy of waveform and pressure reading
  - maintain system and device integrity
  - minimize infection risk

Perform neurological assessment every hour and PRN

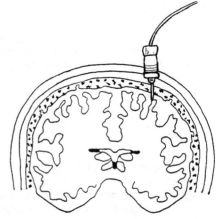

Figure 7.24 Intraparenchymal Monitoring System

Classic Waveforms

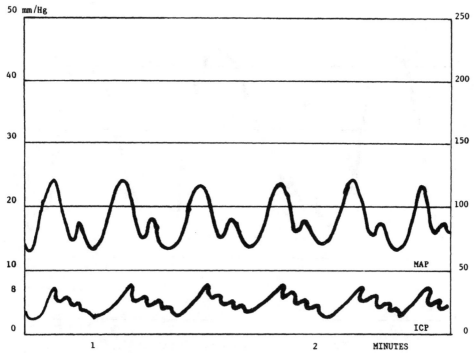

Figure 7.25A Normal ICP Waveform: 4–15 mm/Hg. Normal Arterial Waveform: Systolic, 120; Diastolic, 60; MAP, 80; ICP, 8; CPP, 72

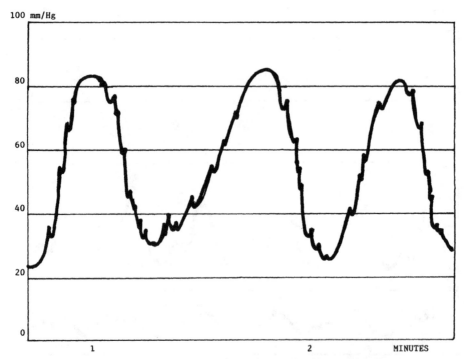

Figure 7.25B   A Waves (Plateau Waves): 50–100 mm/Hg

- Rapid, dangerous rise in ICP
- Decreased ability to compensate
- Sustained = irreversible brain damage

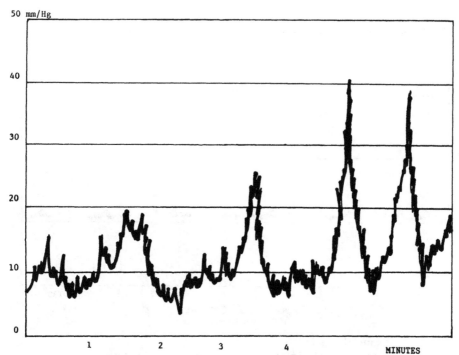

Figure 7.25C　B Waves (Sawtooth Pattern): Frequency, 1–2 min; Up to 50 mm/Hg (Unsustained)

• Possibly decreasing compensation

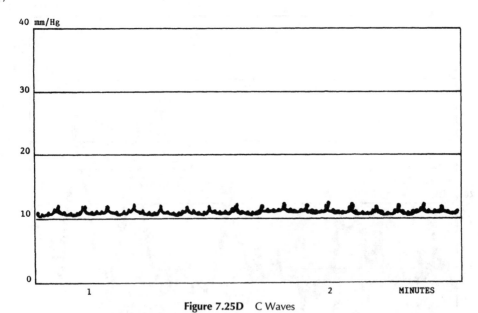

Figure 7.25D C Waves

- Rapid rhythmic
- May fluctuate with respirations or changes in blood pressure
- Usually insignificant

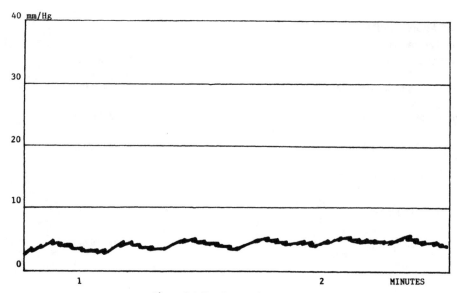

Figure 7.25E   Damped Waveform

- Low, inaccurate reading
- Possible causes: collapse of ventricle
  occlusion of subarachnoid bolt
  kink in pressure tubing

PHYSIOLOGIC MONITORING
Hemodynamic Parameters
Parameter/Formula

Normal Range

Heart rate (HR) = beats/min

60–100 beats/min

Cardiac output (CO) = HR × stroke volume (SV)

4.0–8.0 L/min

$$\text{Cardiac index (CI)} = \frac{CO}{BSA^\dagger}$$

2.5–4.0 L/min/M^2

$$\text{Stroke volume (SV)} = \frac{CO \times 1000 \text{ ml}}{HR}$$

60–100 mL/beat

$$\text{Stroke volume index (SVI)} = \frac{CO \times 1000 \text{ ml}}{BSA \times HR}$$

33–47 mL/beat/M^2

$$\text{Stroke index (SI)} = \frac{CI}{HR} \times 1000$$

30–65 mL/M/beat

Arterial pressure:

$$\text{Mean arterial pressure (MAP)} = \frac{1}{3} \text{ (systolic – diastolic pressure} + \text{diastolic pressure)}$$

Peak systolic 90–140 mm Hg
End diastolic 60–90 mm Hg
Mean 70–100 mm Hg

$$\text{Systemic vascular resistance (SVR)} = \frac{(MAP - RAP) \times 80}{CO}$$

800–1200 dyne/sec/cm^{-5}

$$\text{Left ventricular stroke work index (LVSWI)} = SVI(MAP - PAW) \times 0.0136$$

45–75 gm M/M^2/beat

$\dagger$To calculate body surface area (BSA), see formula p. 309

Pulmonary vascular resistance (PVR) = $\dfrac{(PA - PAW) \times 80}{CO}$

250 dyne/sec/cm^{-5}

Rate–pressure product (RPP) = HR × systolic B/P

12,000

Coronary perfusion pressure = diastolic B/P – PAW

60–70 mm Hg

PA = pulmonary artery

Systolic 17–32 mm Hg
End diastolic 4–13 mm Hg
Mean 9–19 mm Hg

PAWP = pulmonary artery wedge pressure

Mean 4–12 mm Hg

RAP = right atrial pressure

Mean 1–7 mm Hg

RVP = right ventricular pressure

Systolic 17–32 mm Hg
Diastolic 1–7 mm Hg

RVEDP = right ventricular end diastolic pressure

2–6 mm Hg

Right ventricular stroke work index (RVSWI) = (PAM – CVP) SVI × 0.136

8.5–12 g/m^2/beat

Ejection fraction (EF) = $\dfrac{SV}{\text{end diastrolic volume}} \times 100$

60%

Parameter/Formula	*Normal Range*
Rate pressure product = HR × SBP	<12,000
Arterial oxygen content (CaO_2) = $(SaO_2 × Hb × 1.38) + (PaO_2 × 0.0031)$	18–20 ml/100 ml or vol %
Venous oxygen content (CvO_2) = $(SvO_2 × Hb × 1.38) + (PvO_2 × 0.0031)$	15.5 ml/100 ml or vol %
Arterial venous oxygen content difference = $CaO_2 − CvO_2$	4–6 ml/100 ml or vol %
Arterial oxygen delivery (DO_2) = $CO × 10 × CaO_2$	900–1200 ml/min
SVO_2 = O_2 saturation of venous blood	60%–80%

Respiratory Quotients

Venous oxygen delivery (DO_2) = $CO × 10 × CvO_2$	775 ml/min
Oxygen consumption (VO_2) = $CO × 10 × CO_2 (a − v)$	200–250 ml/min
Mixed venous oxygen saturation (SvO_2) = $1 − VO_2/DO_2$	60%–80%
Alveolar-arterial oxygen gradient $(AaDO_2)$ = $PAO_2 − PaO_2$	<15 mm Hg
Alveolar partial pressure of oxygen (PAO_2) = $FIO_2 − PaCO_2$	0.8
Respiratory quotient (RQ) = $\dfrac{O_2 \text{ consumption}}{CO_2 \text{ production}}$	0.8–1

Neurologic Parameters

Cerebral perfusion pressure (CPP) = MAP − ICP   80–100 mm Hg

Intracranial pressure (ICP)   0–15 mm Hg

Renal Parameters

Anion gap (GAP) = Na − (HCO$_3$ + Cl)   8–16 mEq/L

Osmolality (OSM) = (2Na) + K + BUN/3 + Glucose/18   275–295 mOsm

Glomerular filtration rate (GRF) = $\dfrac{140 - \text{Age}) \times \text{wt (kg)}}{\text{(male) } 75 \times \text{serum Cr}}$ 80–120 ml/min

(female) 85 × serum Cr

MONITORING HEMODYNAMIC PARAMETERS
Arterial Pressure Monitoring
When setting up an arterial pressure monitoring system follow the directions provided by the manufacturer. Comply with all hospital policies and procedures that apply to the process.

Indications
- Accurate B/P determination
  - hemodynamic instability
  - titration of vasoactive/inotropic medication
- Assessment of aortic valve closure, perfusion of ectopic beats, and cardiac contraction
- Arterial blood gas sampling
- Lab sampling

Contraindications
- Bleeding dyscrasias
- During use of thrombolytic agents, if an A-line is to be used, it must be placed prior to beginning therapy; insertion site must be monitored closely for signs of bleeding; if necessary to remove line after therapy is begun, *manual* pressure must be held on the site for *30* min

Complications
- Accidental blood loss
- Compromised flow to extremity
- Sepsis
- Dissection of involved artery
- Air embolism
- Hematoma
- Thrombosis
- Arterial spasms

Components
- Heparinized flush solution
  - mix according to hospital policy
- Micro drip administration set (60 gtt/cc)
- Pressure tubing
- Continuous flush device with three-way stopcock
- Two-way stopcock
- Pressure transducer
- Transducer mounting bracket
- Pressure infusor bag
- Cannula
- Transducer interface cable
- Electronic monitoring system

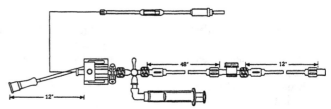

Figure 7.26 Disposable Pressure Monitoring Kit and Safedraw Closed-Loop Blood Sampling System

Reprinted with permission of Ohmeda, Inc. (Madison, WI), 1995.

Nursing/Medical Implications
- Most common sites for arterial cannulation are radial, brachial, and femoral; dorsalis pedis also may be used
- Less frequently used sites include axillary and temporal arteries and umbilical artery in neonate
- Cannulation of artery is a sterile technique
- All equipment should be assembled, flushed, zeroed, and calibrated before cannulation is attempted
- Prior to cannulating the artery, Allen's test should be performed to ascertain that there is adequate collateral circulation to the hand
  - ulnar *and* radial arteries should be occluded by manual pressure
  - patient should clench and unclench fist until hand blanches (approximately 1 min)
  - release pressure on ulnar artery only
  - observe for return of color to hand
    - ulnar circulation is adequate if color returns to hand within 5–7 sec

- – ulnar filling considered impaired if color takes 7–15 sec to return to normal. This is an *absolute* contraindication for placement of an arterial catheter.
  - – if hand remains blanched for longer than 15 sec, ulnar circulation is considered inadequate and radial artery should not be cannulated
- Indwelling arterial catheter pressures are more accurate in low-flow states than those obtained by indirect auscultation
- Arterial line pressures normally 5–20 mm Hg higher than auscultated pressure
- Pressure valves obtained from an arterial line should be compared with auscultated pressures at least every 8 hr and when there is doubt as to accuracy of arterial line pressure
- Insertion sites should be monitored closely for signs of infection; system integrity should never be breached
- All connections in system should be kept securely closed to prevent accidental blood loss or air embolus
- Dressing, tubing, and flush solution changes should be done in compliance with institutional policies and procedures
- Extremity involved should be immobilized and visible
- Insertion site and connections must be easily accessible
- Maintain sterility of all ports and caps when obtaining blood samples
- High and low pressure limits must be set appropriately for each patient and alarms must be activated
- Circulation to extremity involved should be monitored continuously
- Impaired circulation should be reported immediately; removal of device may be necessary
- Zero and calibrate transducer every 8 hr and as needed
  - – to zero system
    - – place transducer at zero reference point (right atrial level)
    - – turn stopcock nearest transducer *off to the patient;* transducer then is open to air; proceed with calibration as appropriate to the system in use, complying with institutional policies and procedures
- Maintain transducer at a consistent level when taking readings

Characteristics of the Waveform

- Normal
  - *upstroke:* rapid ejection phase
    - indicates stroke volume; sloped upstroke may indicate reduced stroke volume
  - *dicrotic notch* on downstroke indicates
    - aortic valve closure
    - termination of ventricular systole
  - *anacrotic notch* at end diastole indicates
    - diminishing pressure in arterial system
- Arterial waveform with resonance
  - resonance artifact can be produced by under-damped tubing system; reflects
    - length and stiffness of pressure tubing
    - compliance of transducer dome, stopcocks, flush device
    - air bubbles
  - R.O.S.E.® (resonance overshoot eliminator): a device engineered to eliminate systolic overshoot caused by underdamping in pressure monitoring systems
    - calibrated to provide optimum damping without adjustments
    - totally closed design

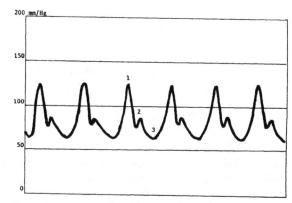

Figure 7.27   Normal A-Line Waveform: 1 = Systolic Peak (90–140 mm Hg); 2 = Diacrotic Notch; 3 = End-Diastolic (60–90 mm Hg); Mean Arterial Pressure = 70–100 mm Hg

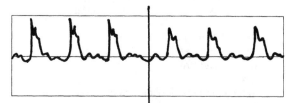

Figure 7.28   Resonance Overshoot Artifact Without R.O.S.E.® *(left);* Resonance Overshoot Artifact With R.O.S.E.® *(right)*

– isolated air chamber
– air and bacteria prevented from entering system
– no risk of bleed back
– requires no extra setup or fluid filling procedures

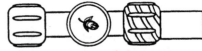

Figure 7.29   R.O.S.E.® Resonance Over-shoot Eliminator

Reprinted with permission of Ohmeda, Inc. (Madison, WI), 1995.

Arterial Pressure Values
• Normal
  – systolic: 90–140 mm Hg
  – diastolic: 60–90 mm Hg
  – mean: 70–100 mm Hg

Physiological/Technical Reasons for Variance in Arterial Pressure Values

Physiological (High Values)	*Physiological (Low Values)*	*Technical (High Values)*	*Technical (Low Values)*
• Increased peripheral resistance	• Low peripheral resistance	• Zero level too low	• Zero level too high
• Systemic hypertension	• Decreased cardiac output	• Catheter too small	• Vasospasm
• Aortic insufficiency	• Aortic stenosis	• Catheter "fling" or "whip"	• Damped line caused by air bubbles, fibrin clots, or excessively long pressure line
• Arteriosclerosis		• Resonance	

Evaluation of Abnormal Waveforms
• Normal tracing (see Figure 7.27, p. 277)
• Damped waveform
  – cause
    – catheter may be lodged against arterial wall
    – fibrin clots on tip of catheter

- appearance
  - slow upstroke
  - flattened waveform
  - narrow pulse pressure
  - indiscernible dicrotic notch
- Bigeminal pulse (may be confused with pulsus alternans)
  - cause
    - occurrence of premature contractions, usually ventricular, every other beat
  - appearance
    - irregular rhythm with smaller premature beat following shorter interval
- Pulsus alternans (may be confused with pulsus bigeminus)
  - cause
    - left ventricular failure
    - may be precipitated by PVC
  - appearance
    - regular rhythm
    - size and intensity of pulses vary
- Pulsus bisferiens
  - cause
    - aortic insufficiency
    - aortic stenosis with insufficiency
    - hypertrophic obstructed cardiomyopathy

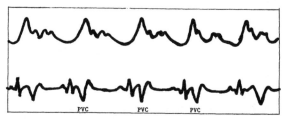

Figure 7.30   Bigeminal Pulse

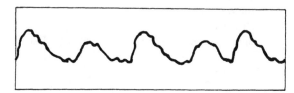

Figure 7.31   Pulsus Alternans

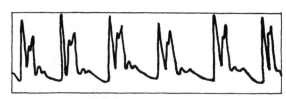

Figure 7.32   Pulsus Bisferiens

- appearance
  - bifid systolic peaks
  - peaks may be equal or either may be larger than the other
- Pulsus paradoxus
  - causes
    - cardiac tamponade
    - chronic constrictive pericarditis
    - severe emphysema, bronchial asthma
    - hypovolemic shock
    - pulmonary embolus
    - extreme obesity
    - patient on positive pressure mechanical ventilation
  - appearance
    - during spontaneous inspiration, amplitude of pulse waveform decreases more than the usual 10 mm Hg or less

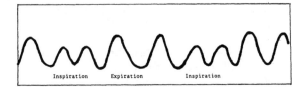

Figure 7.33   Pulsus Paradoxus

Multilumen Central Venous Catheter
This device allows simultaneous, separate access by means of a single insertion site. Insertion and maintenance techniques should comply with institutional policies and protocols.

Indications
- Unavailable peripheral access
- Conditions necessitating long-term access
- Trauma, burns
- High-risk surgery
- Cardiovascular surgery
- Acute MI
- Poor nutritional status, dehydration

Contraindications
- Preexisting sepsis
- Known heparin sensitivity

Advantages
- Fluid/medication administration (continuous/intermittent)
- Administration of blood or blood products
- TPN
- Concurrent administration of incompatible medications
- Venous blood sampling
- Central venous pressure monitoring
- Chemotherapy
- Prevents loss of peripheral vein to caustic, erosive, or painful drug therapy
- Reduces necessity for repeated venipuncture

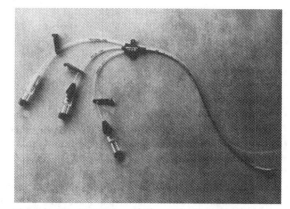

Figure 7.34 ARROWguard Blue Multi-Lumen Catheter

Reprinted with permission of Arrow International, Inc. (Reading, PA), 1995.

Complications
- Bleeding
- Catheter disengagement/occlusion
- Infection/sepsis
- Thrombus formation
- Embolus
- Cardiac perforation
- Pneumothorax

Nursing/Medical Implications
- Suggested insertion sites: internal jugular vein or subclavian vein
- Chest film should be done to verify catheter placement in superior vena cava
- Distal tip of catheter should not be placed in right atrium
- Lumens may be kept patent by continuous infusion with heparin solutions, heparin lock, or intermittent flush
- Distal lumen should be utilized to obtain CVP
- If catheter cannot be aspirated or irrigated, do not attempt to force; verify that catheter is not kinked; if occlusion cannot be resolved, clamp lumen and notify physician
- Urokinase (5000 I.U./mL) may be used to declot an occluded catheter

Physician must perform declotting procedure.

Recommended Lumen Usage

Lumen	Function
Proximal (18 ga)	• Fluid administration
	• Medication administration
	• Blood sampling
Middle (18 ga)	• Fluid administration
	• Medication administration if TPN not anticipated during life of catheter
	• Hyperalimentation

Distal (16 ga)	• Fluid administration
	• Medication administration
	• Blood and blood products
	• High-volume fluid administration
	• Colloids
	• Blood sampling
	• CVP monitoring

Central Venous Pressure (CVP) Monitoring
Right atrial pressure is a reflection of right ventricular end diastolic pressure (RVEDP)

Normal Valve
- 5–12 cm H_2O or 4–11 mm Hg

Indications
- Determination of fluid volume status by measurement of pressures in vena cava and right atrium
- Evaluation of heart as an effective pump
- Assessment of vascular tension quality
- Reflection of preload

Complications
- Line displacement
- Line disconnection
- Air embolus
- Thrombosis
- Infection/sepsis
- Ischemia of involved limb

Monitoring Technique

- Readings obtained in cm H_2O
  - catheter threaded into vena cava via peripheral or subclavian vein
  - a manometer with three-way stopcock placed between fluid source and catheter
  - three fluid pathways created
    - pathway 1 connects fluid source to patient, facilitating intravenous fluid administration
    - pathway 2 connects fluid source to CVP manometer; stopcock is opened and fluid in column rises prior to pressure measurement
    - pathway 3 connects intravenous catheter to manometer; when pathway is open, pressure in vena cava equilibrates with pressure in fluid column; CVP recorded when fluid level settles at a given point
- Readings obtained in mm Hg per pressure transducer
  - Measured via PA (intracardiac) catheter
  - *proximal lumen* of PA catheter connected to transducer and monitor
  - to obtain CVP reading, follow manufacturer's directions unique to system used
  - if fluids are administered through proximal port of PA catheter, system should be calibrated prior to obtaining CVP reading

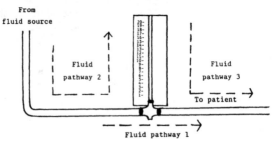

Figure 7.35   CVP Manometer

Variations in CVP Readings

- *High readings* produced by
  - CHF
  - cardiac tamponade
  - increased blood volume (overtransfusion or overhydration)
  - vasoconstriction
  - tricuspid valve dysfunction
  - right ventricular dysfunction (>15 cm H_2O)
  - left ventricular dysfunction (>18 mm Hg)
  - constrictive pericarditis
  - pulmonary hypertension
- *Low readings* produced by
  - hypovolemia (blood loss, diuresis)
  - vasodilation (drug induced)
  - decreased venous tone
  - peripheral blood pooling

Nursing/Medical Implications

- CVP may be measured either in cm H_2O or mm Hg by using a pressure transducer
- Pressures obtained by these methods vary considerably
  - right atrium pressure is 0–4 cm H_2O
  - vena cava pressure is approximately 6–12 cm H_2O
  - right atrial pressure per pressure transducer is 3–11 mm Hg
- Trend of CVP values is more important than isolated reading
- CVP readings are most valuable when interpreted in conjunction with other available hemodynamic parameters and clinical assessments
- For accurate measurement, patient should be flat and zero point of manometer at level of the phlebostatic axis, zero reference point (at the 4th ICS approximately 5 cm below sternum, midaxilla)

- If patient is *absolutely* unable to lie flat, readings may be taken in semi-Fowler's position, but must be done consistently and documented
- Readings may be falsely high if patient is on a ventilator
- Hospital protocol or physician requests should be complied with in determining whether patient is to be removed from ventilator during CVP readings; trends should be observed as long as readings are obtained consistently, either on or off the ventilator

Intracardiac Catheters

Because each manufacturer of intracardiac catheters has unique guidelines for use, refer to product information prior to initiating therapy. During catheter insertion, emergency drugs, defibrillation equipment, and respiratory assistance equipment should be at hand.

Devices for measuring intracardiac pressures range from a single-lumen pulmonary artery pressure (PAP) catheter to sophisticated catheters that measure continuous SVO_2 readings. Additionally, a catheter may have a right ventricular lumen through which a pacing probe may be inserted. There is also available a Swan–Ganz® thermodilution catheter that is capable of atrial and ventricular pacing, AV sequential pacing, intraatrial and intraventricular EKG monitoring.[†]

Indications
- Requirement of rapid hemodynamic assessment in situations of
  - MI
  - shock
  - CHF
  - coronary artery bypass surgery
  - vascular surgery
  - pulmonary edema/embolism
  - respiratory failure/mechanical ventilation
  - circulating assistance device (IABP)
  - hemodialysis
  - cardiac tamponade/effusion

- Blood sampling
- Fluid management

Contraindications

- Bleeding disorders (especially thrombocytopenia)
- Thrombolytic therapy
- Immunosuppression (severely compromised host)
- Terminal disease states
- Lack of appropriately trained personnel

Advantages

- Permits precise pressure monitoring even when patient is in shock
- More accurate than noninvasive monitoring methods
- Rapidly identifies subtle changes in cardiovascular status
- Reflects patient response to therapeutic intervention; intropic/vasoactive drugs, diuretics, and administration of fluids

Disadvantages

- Increased risk of complications
  - bleeding
  - embolus
  - infection/sepsis
  - cardiac dysrhythmias (PACs/PVCs)
  - pulmonary artery perforation
  - pulmonary infarction
  - pneumothorax
  - endocarditis
- Requires specialized training in identifying and interpreting hemodynamic parameters and/or equipment malfunction

- May foster false sense of security; *must* be remembered that machines only augment astute clinical observations
- Looping of catheter in right atrium or right ventricle

Nursing/Medical Implications
- Manipulation of intracardiac catheter must be guided *strictly* by institutional policies and procedures
- Common access sites: subclavian vein, internal jugular vein, median basilic or femoral vein
- Advancement of catheter to pulmonary artery (PA) should be accomplished quickly; prolonged manipulation may result in increased catheter flexibility, spasm, and difficulty entering PA
- Because it is flow directed, catheter may be inserted at bedside by continuous pressure monitoring; how-ever, fluoroscopy is recommended for femoral inser-tion
- Catheter placement must be ascertained by chest X-ray
- To ascertain that catheter tip is in thorax, have patient cough, which should produce rapid oscilla-tion on pressure monitor of ≥40 mm Hg
- When tip of catheter is in range of right atrium (RA), pressure oscillation on monitor normally is about 3–6 mm Hg (RA in Figure 7.36)
- Range of pressure oscillation greatly increases as catheter tip enters right ventricle (RV) (RV in Figure 7.36); normal range is 17–32 mm Hg/systolic, 1–7 mm Hg/diastolic

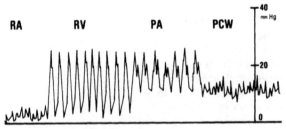

Figure 7.36 Waveforms Produced During Insertion of an Intracardiac Catheter

From Hemodynamic Measurements Made With the Swan–Ganz® Catheter. Reprinted with permission from Baxter Health-care Corporation, Edwards Critical-Care Division, 1987.

- Closely monitor patient's EKG to identify ventricular ectopy, which may occur as catheter tip passes through tricuspid valve
- As catheter enters PA, look for marked increase in diastolic pressure; peak systolic pressure should not change from that noted in RV reading; normal range is 17–32 mm Hg/systolic, 4–13 mm Hg/end diastolic, and mean 9–19 mm Hg (PA in Figure 7.36)
- With proper wedging, oscillation range is approximately 2 mm Hg and closely approximates PA diastolic pressure if there is no significant lung disease
- Wedge readings should be done per physician order; pulmonary artery wedge pressure (PAWP) readings usually not ordered more frequently than every 4 hr; balloon may rupture if inflated more frequently
- Mean pulmonary artery wedge pressure (4–12 mm Hg) should be 1–4 mm Hg *less* than pulmonary artery diastolic pressure
- If 15 cm PEEP, falsely elevated PCWP is likely. Formula to calculate "true" PCWP:

$$\text{true wedge} = \text{measured PCWP} - \frac{(\text{PEEP level})\ 0.75}{2}$$

- PAP reflects pulmonary venous pressure as well as mean filling pressure for left side of heart; PA systolic pressure usually equals RV systolic pressure unless there is pulmonary stenosis; PAP reflects right ventricular function
- A rise in PAP may indicate
  - pulmonary hypertension
  - increased pulmonary blood flow
  - mitral stenosis
  - left ventricular failure
  - fluid overload
- Catheter tip migration must be recognized as a potential danger; pulmonary infarction may result if catheter migrates to wedge position while balloon is deflated

- Catheter tip may migrate into RV; when this occurs, diastolic pressure drops into range of mean RA pressure; attempt should be made to advance the catheter tip to PA; when this cannot be accomplished, catheter replacement may be necessary
- When withdrawing catheter, balloon must be *deflated* to preclude damage when passing through heart valves
- Pressure damping may occur and should be recognized early so that appropriate interventions may be instituted to correct the situation
  - kinking of a lumen: inspect tubing and ensure that kinks are straightened and flush solution is unimpeded
  - air bubbles in catheter lumen, transducer, or stopcock: when setting up system, carefully flush transducer and tubing; inspect for bubbles before attaching catheter; check connections frequently for patency
  - most frequent cause of pressure damping is a clot in catheter lumen: an attempt may be made to aspirate the clot; if clot is removed, flush system with heparinized solution by using fast-flush valve; *never* flush a hemodynamic line with a syringe
  - catheter wedged against vessel wall: make sure that balloon is completely deflated; have patient cough and fast flush the catheter
  - too high or too low, not zeroed: level transducer with patient's right atrium and zero to atmospheric pressure
- If catheter wedges at a volume significantly less than expected maximum, catheter tip is probably too far advanced in the pulmonary circulation; balloon should be deflated and catheter repositioned

Catheter
Two lumens

Function
- Distal port for PAP and PAWP monitoring
- Balloon inflation port

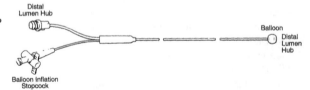

Figure 7.37   CritiCath® Two-Lumen Catheter
Reprinted with permission of Ohmeda, Inc., 1995.

Three lumens

- Distal port for PAP and PAWP monitoring
- Proximal port for RA (CVP) pressure monitoring/IV medication, etc., only
- Balloon inflation port

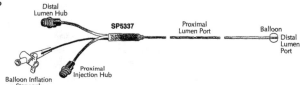

Figure 7.38 CritiCath® Three-Lumen Catheter
Reprinted with permission of Ohmeda, Inc., 1995.

CritiCath®
four-lumen
thermodilution
catheter

- Distal port for PAP and PAWP monitoring. Blood samples may be obtained from this lumen for mixed venous studies
- Proximal port for RA (CVP) pressure monitoring; IV infusion/medication administration; carries injectate solution to right atrium for CO
- Balloon inflation port
- Thermistor and computer connector cable for thermodilution CO measurement

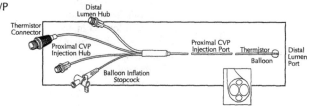

Figure 7.39 CritiCath® Four-Lumen Thermodilution Catheter
Reprinted with permission of Ohmeda, Inc., 1995.

Catheter
CritiCath®
five-lumen
thermodilution
catheter

Function
- Same as four-lumen device, plus
  – a proximal medication lumen, which may be used to measure right atrial pressure, carry injectate solution to the right atrium for cardiac output, blood sampling, and drug administration

The CritiCath® five-lumen catheter also is available with a right ventricular lumen. This lumen should *not* be used for CO injectate; it facilitates blood sampling, drug infusion, and right ventricular pressure monitoring.

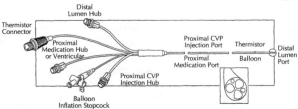

Figure 7.40 CritiCath® Five-Lumen Thermodilution Catheter
Reprinted with permission of Ohmeda, Inc., 1995.

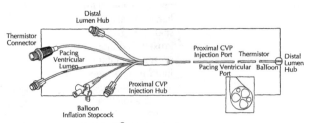

Figure 7.41 CritiCath® Pacing Catheter
Reprinted with permission of Ohmeda, Inc., 1995.

CritiCath®
pacing catheter

- Same as the four-lumen device, plus
  – a lumen that accommodates a pacing probe

Swan–Ganz®
A-V Paceport™
Thermodilution
Catheter

- Full hemodynamic monitoring
- Temporary ⟩ with Flex-Tip™
  - atrial pacing ⟩ transluminal
  - AV pacing ⟋ A-Pacing probe
  - ventricular pacing with Chandler™
    transluminal V-Pacing probe
- Intra-atrial EKG monitoring
- Intra-ventricular EKG monitoring
- Distal port (RV)
  - color-coded orange
  - ventricular pacing
- Proximal port (RA)
  - color-coded yellow
  - atrial pacing
  - fluid infusion
- Balloon inflation port
- Blood sampling from right ventricular
  lumen when pacing probe is not inserted

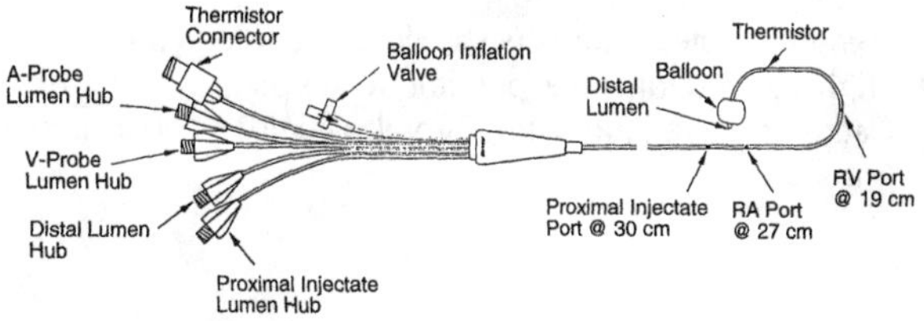

Figure 7.42 Swan–Ganz® A-V Paceport™ Thermodilution Catheter

Reprinted with permission of Baxter Healthcare Corporation (Santa Ana, CA), 1995.

Contraindications
- Pacemaker-dependent patients
- Recurrent/active sepsis
- Clotting dyscrasia that tends to thrombus formation

Thromboshield™ catheters are contraindicated for any patients with known heparin sensitivity.

Complications
- Cardiac dysrhythmias
- Tricuspid/pulmonic valve damage
- Perforation of pulmonary artery
- Pulmonary infarction
- Pneumothorax
- Cardiac tamponade
- Thrombus
- Catheter knotting
- Sepsis/infection (endocarditis)
- Thrombocytopenia
- Stimulation of the diaphragm

Nursing/Medical Implications
- Catheter is flow directed
- Heparin-coated catheters should be handled cautiously to preclude removal of anticoagulant
- High-volume infusions possible when pacing probe *not* in place
- Catheter is available with Thromboshield™ heparin coating; catheters so protected have an "H" in the model number

Catheter
Baxter REF-1™
(right-ejection
fraction)*

Function
- Cardiac output
- PA and wedge pressures
- Right ventricular
  - ejection fraction
  - stroke volume
  - end diastolic volume
- Heart rate
- Indices
  - cardiac index
  - stroke volume index
  - right ventricular end diastolic volume index
  - right ventricular end stroke volume index

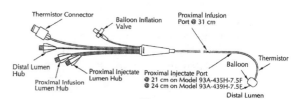

Figure 7.43A Baxter REF-1™ Catheter

Reprinted with permission of Baxter Healthcare Corporation (Santa Ana, CA), 1995.

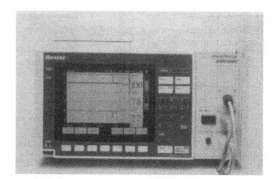

Figure 7.43B REF-1™ Computer Explorer® Monitor

Reprinted with permission of Baxter Healthcare Corporation (Santa Ana, CA), 1995.

---

*Used with dedicated REF-1 computer that measures ejection fraction and cardiac output (see Figure 7.43B). Compatible with all other Swan-Ganz® thermodilution catheters for purposes of cardiac output.

Indications

- Increased pulmonary vascular resistance
  - pulmonary disease
  - pulmonary hypertension
  - pulmonary embolus
  - sepsis
  - PEEP/mechanical ventilation
- Right ventricular dysfunction
  - pulmonary diseases
  - blunt chest trauma
  - right ventricular infarct
  - right ventricular heart failure
- Left ventricular dysfunction
  - mitral stenosis
  - acute mitral valve regurgitation
  - left ventricular infarct
  - left ventricular heart failure
  - cardiogenic shock
- Volume disturbances
  - fluid imbalance
  - fluid resuscitation
  - burn patients
- Major surgical procedures
  - thoracic surgery
  - coronary bypass
  - transplant surgery

CONTINUOUS CARDIAC OUTPUT/SVO$_2$ MONITORING

Continuous cardiac output monitoring improves on the intermittent measurements of the bolus technique by way of a thermal filament placed in the right heart. Moment-to-moment data allows the clinician to track subtle changes in the cardiovascular system. The Baxter IntelliCath™ and Vigilance® monitor system constantly evaluates temperature of the thermal filament and provides crucial clues to cardiovascular status. The CCOmbo™ catheter performs these functions and, additionally, provides continuous SVO$_2$ measurements. The Vigilance® monitor is compatible with Swan–Ganz® catheters for purposes of measuring cardiac output via bolus thermodilution.

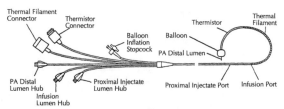

Figure 7.44 Baxter IntelliCath™ Catheter

Reprinted with permission of Baxter Healthcare Corporation (Santa Ana, CA), 1995.

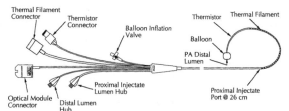

Figure 7.45 Baxter CCOmbo™ Catheter

Reprinted with permission of Baxter Healthcare Corporation (Santa Ana, CA), 1995.

Interpretation of Variations in SVO$_2$

SVO$_2$ Reading	Variation	Etiology
60%–80% (Normal)	• Oxygen delivery = oxygen demand	• Perfusion adequate
<60% (Low)	• Decreased oxygen delivery	• Hypoperfusion
		• Decreased CO
		• Hypoxemia
		• Anemia, hemorrhage
		• Hypoxia, suctioning
	• Increased oxygen consumption	• Activity/exercise
		• Seizures
		• Shivering
		• Pain
		• Hyperthermia
		• Anxiety
80%–95% (High)	• Increased oxygen delivery	• Increased oxygen in tissues and organs
	• Mechanical interference	• PA catheter wedged
		• Left to right shunt
	• Decreased oxygen consumption	• Anesthesia
		• Sepsis
		• Hypothermia
		• Paralysis induced by pharmacologic agents

Nursing/Medical Implications
- Determinants of oxygen transport
  - CO
  - arterial oxygenation
  - hemoglobin
- When preparing catheter for insertion, avoid bending so as to prevent damage to optical fibers

- Insertion site chosen at physician's discretion; internal jugular and subclavian routes are frequently used; anticubital vein is safe, but placement may be difficult without fluoroscopy; movement of patient's arm also may cause manipulation of catheter
- When attempting PA catheter placement in a patient with LBBB, use of catheter with pacing capabilities may be expedient
- Oximeter should be calibrated daily, with a blood sample of known oxygen saturation, according to manufacturer's instructions; machine also should be calibrated if readings are inexplicably deranged
- Balloon should be inflated as infrequently as practical; monitor, instead, pulmonary artery end-diastolic pressure (PAEDP)
- Coiling or knotting of catheter usually associated with prolonged insertion time
- During insertion, if catheter becomes flexible and difficult to advance, it may be flushed with iced saline or an appropriate guide wire may be used

Hemodynamic Subsets of Acute Myocardial Infarction

	Indications	PAW	Therapy	Mortality
Subset I No failure	Cardiac index >2.2 L/min/ M^2	<18 mm Hg	Sedate	3%
Subset II Pulmonary congestion	Cardiac index >2.2 L/min/ M^2	>18 mm Hg	Normal blood pressure: diuretics; elevated blood pressure: vasodilators	9%
Subset III Peripheral hypoperfusion	Cardiac index <2.2 L/min/ M^2	<18 mm Hg	Elevated heart rate: add volume; depressed heart rate: pacing	23%
Subset IV Congestion and hypoperfusion	Cardiac index <2.2 L/min/ M^2	>18 mm Hg	Depressed blood pressure: inotropes; normal blood pressure: vasodilators	51%

Reprinted with permission of James S. Forrester, M.D., Assistant Director of Cardiology, Cedars-Sinai Medical Center, Los Angeles, California.

EPIDURAL CATHETER

Indications
- Postoperative pain relief
- Management of pain intractable to other methods of control
- Anesthesia for surgery of lower abdomen, inguinal area, lower extremities
- Obstetrical, gynecological procedures
- Airway abnormalities precluding general anesthesia

Contraindications
- Previous difficulty with spinal anesthesia
- Backache
- Preoperative use of anticoagulant
- Neurological deficit
- Infections of the back
- Prolonged operative procedure

Advantages
- Prolonged pain control (6–24 hr)
- Reduces narcotic requirements
- Earlier mobility postoperatively
- Minimizes narcotic administration side effects

Disadvantages
- Urinary retention
- Respiratory depression
- Pruritis
- Nausea, vomiting
- Possible postural hypotension

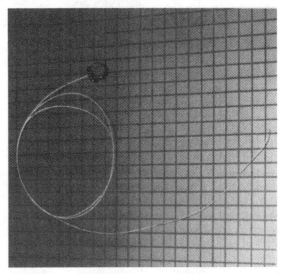

Figure 7.46   Epidural Catheter

Reprinted with permission of Kendall Healthcare Products Co., 1995.

Complications
- Bleeding, irritation at the exit site
- Infection
- Occluded catheter
- Catheter malposition
- Disconnection of system components
- Pain on injection
- Inadequate pain relief

Nursing/Medical Implications
- Careful differentiation between nursing and medical responsibilities must be outlined
- Respiratory rate must be carefully monitored *during* and for 6–24 hr after epidural narcotic is discontinued
- An apnea monitor may be used
- Emergency equipment should be readily available
- Use a 0.22-μ filter on the catheter to prevent particulate matter or bacteria from entering epidural space
- Naloxone (Narcan) must be kept at hand when catheter is being used for pain management
- Only preservative-free narcotics should be injected into catheter
- When epidural narcotics are in use, parenteral narcotics must be withheld until anesthesiologist is consulted
- Parenteral narcotics should not be administered for 6–24 hr after epidural injections have been discontinued
- Epidural pain control may be managed intermittently (by anesthesiologist) or regulated by controlled delivery system
- No other drugs may be injected via this route
- Strict aseptic technique required when caring for epidural line
- *Only* the anesthesiologist may institute or discontinue an epidural catheter
- Frequent assessments of motor function level are a responsibility of the nurse
- Nurses must be knowledgeable of drugs administered by an epidural catheter (usually morphine or fentanyl)
- Alcohol should not be used during site care as it may migrate along the catheter and could cause neurological damage; povidone–iodine solution should be used

ROTATING TOURNIQUETS

Functions
- Decreases circulating volume
- Decreases venous return to heart

Indications
- Severe CHF
- Acute pulmonary edema

Complications
- May cause hypotension
- Circulatory overload if cuffs are removed too quickly
- Peripheral ischemia
- Skin breakdown
- Cardiorespiratory arrest

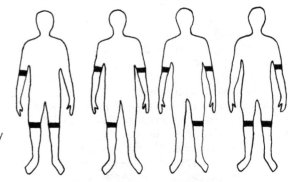

Figure 7.47   Rotating Tourniquets

Nursing/Medical Implications
- Obtain baseline BP reading before instituting rotating tourniquets
- Cuff should be placed high on extremity
- Cuff pressure should be maintained just above the patient's diastolic pressure
- Arterial supply to extremity must be maintained
- No cuff should remain inflated longer than 45 min
- When therapy is discontinued, cuffs should be removed in rotating sequence, one every 15 min, allowing blood to return gradually to systemic circulation
- Automatic devices are available; may also be performed manually
- Emergency equipment should be close at hand during use of rotating tourniquets
- While using tourniquets, keep a flow sheet to maintain continuity

MEDICAL ANTISHOCK TROUSERS (MAST) AND PNEUMATIC ANTISHOCK GARMENT (PASG)

Once applied, MAST pressure should not be lowered. Deflation of the device before fluid resuscitation may cause irreversible shock.

Functions
- Increases systemic vascular resistance by translocation of circulating blood
- Prevents shock from blood loss by
  - creating artificial peripheral resistance
  - ensuring adequate coronary artery perfusion
- Elevates B/P in patients with marked hypovolemia
- Reduces potential spaces where hematomas may form
- Increases availability of blood volume to support vital organs

Indications
- Systolic pressure <80 mm Hg
- Trauma
  - fracture of femur or pelvis (fracture of tibia and/or fibula should be managed by a device that immobilizes the ankle; therefore MAST is contraindicated in this case)
- Nontraumatic incidents
  - ruptured abdominal aneurysm
  - vaginal hemorrhage
  - gynecologic hemorrhage (ruptured ectopic pregnancy, uterine hemorrhage)
- Intra-abdominal hemorrhage

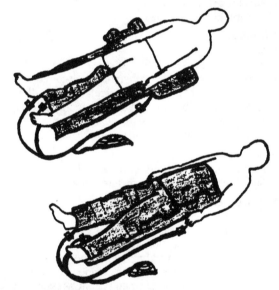

Figure 7.48 Pneumatic Antishock Garment (PASG)

303

Contraindications
- Pulmonary edema
- Cardiogenic shock
- Intrathoracic hemorrhage
- Diaphragmatic rupture
- Tension pneumothorax

Advantages
- Easy, safe application
- Automatic release valves
- Allows patient transfer with minimal discomfort
- Temporarily stabilizes cardiovascular system allowing for controlled fluid therapy and in-depth assessment
- Useful in immobilizing and stabilizing musculoskeletal injuries of lower extremities
- New modular units allow removal of any given component
- New transparent models allow observation and evaluation of injury sites and skin conditions

Disadvantages
- MAST is meant for short-term use; fluid resuscitation should be initiated as quickly as practical
- Significant alterations in pressures may occur with changes in temperature or altitude

Nursing/Medical Implications
- Deflation procedure
  - reduce pressure slowly, beginning with abdominal chamber
  - ascertain that inflation/deflation valves are closed
  - detach foot pump and hose assembly from valves
  - allow small amount of air to escape
  - check blood pressure; when systolic pressure drops 5 mm Hg, cease deflation and infuse IV fluids to return pressure to normal limits

- MAST should not be deflated or removed until
  - a physician has taken charge of patient
  - fluid resuscitation is in progress
  - surgical team/anesthesia is ready for patient, if indicated
- Use of MAST and PASG is controversial; patient requiring this therapy must be monitored closely; *volume resuscitation is imperative;* each section of device must be deflated slowly; fluid and blood must be kept at hand in case of hemodynamic instability when garment is removed
- MAST may be placed directly over open wounds if they have been covered
- Angulated fractures must be straightened and manual traction maintained until MAST is pressurized and splinting is secure
- If severe damage to a limb requires a tourniquet, MAST can be applied if it does not interfere with tourniquet

chapter **8**

DRUGS/CALCULATIONS

CONVERSION

WEIGHTS, MEASURES, AND EQUIVALENTS
Apothecaries' System
Weight
1 scruple (Э) = 20 grains (gr)
1 dram (ʒ) = 60 grains
1 ounce (ʒ) = 480 grains, or 8 drams (dr)
1 pound (lb) = 5760 grains, or 12 ounces (oz)
1 grain = 60 milligrams
1/100 grain = 0.6 milligram
1/150 grain = 0.4 milligram

Metric System
Weight
1 milligram (mg) = 1000 micrograms
1 gram (g/gm) = 1000 milligrams
1 kilogram (Kg) = 1000 grams
1 kilogram = 2.2 pounds

Approximate Equivalents: Linear Measure
1 millimeter (mm) ≅ 0.04 inch (in.)
1 centimeter (cm) ≅ 0.4 inch
1 decimeter (dm) ≅ 4.0 inches
1 meter (m)   ≅ 39.37 inches

Volume
1 fluid dram (ʒ) = 60 minims (m)
1 fluid ounce (ʒ) = 480 minims, or 8 fluid drams
1 pint (pt) = 7680 minims, or 16 fluid ounces
1 quart (qt) = 2 pints
1 gallon (gal) = 4 quarts
1 liter fluid = 1 kilogram

Volume
1 cubic centimeter = 1000 cubic millimeters
1 liter (L) = 1000 cubic centimeters

Approximate Equivalents: Liquid Measure

Metric		Apothecaries'
0.06 mL	≅	1 minim
0.5 mL	≅	8 minims
1.0 mL	≅	15 minims
4.0 mL	≅	1 fluid dram

Metric		Apothecaries'
5 mL	≅	1 teaspoon
15 mL	≅	1 tablespoon
30 mL	≅	1 fluid ounce
250 mL	≅	8 fluid ounces
500 mL	≅	1 pint
1000 mL	≅	1 quart

TEMPERATURE CONVERSION FORMULA

$$C = \frac{5}{9}(F - 32) \qquad\qquad F = \left(C \times \frac{9}{5}\right) + 32$$

CONVERTING mm Hg TO cm H$_2$O (FOR CVP)

To convert mm Hg to cm H$_2$O, multiply mm Hg by 1.34

FORMULA FOR OBTAINING BODY SURFACE AREA (BSA)

$$\text{BSA (m}^2) = \sqrt{\frac{\text{ht (cm)} \times \text{wt (kg)}}{3600}} \text{ or BSA (m}^2) = \sqrt{\frac{\text{ht (in)} \times \text{wt (lb)}}{3131}}$$

Body surface area also may be obtained utilizing the Du Bois BSA normogram.

Modified BSA formula equation by Gehan and George reprinted with permission from *Handbook of Critical Care,* 3rd edition, James Berk and James Sampliner, Eds. Boston: Little, Brown and Company, 1990.

CRITICAL CALCULATIONS

Drug Concentration per mL (cc)

$$\frac{\text{Known amount of drug}}{\text{Total volume of diluent}} = \text{amount of drug/mL (concentration)}$$

Example: $\dfrac{400 \text{ mg dopamine}}{500 \text{ mL D}_5\text{W}} = 0.8 \text{ mg/mL} \quad \text{or} \quad 800 \text{ mcg/mL}$

Dose/Drop (gtt) from Dose/mL

Example: A patient is to receive 800 mcg/mL of dopamine. Because 60 gtt = 1 mL, the concentration may be given at 800 mcg/mL (60 gtt), or 13.3 mcg/gtt.

Dose/Minute from Infusion Rate (IR)

$$\frac{\text{Concentration (dose)} \times \text{infusion rate}}{60 \text{ min}} = \text{dose/min}$$

Example: A patient is to receive 30 gtt/min of a dopamine infusion from a concentration of 400 mg dopamine/500 mL D$_5$W (800 mcg/mL), so

$$\frac{800 \text{ mcg/mL} \times 30 \text{ gtt/min (cc/hr)}}{60 \text{ min}} = 400 \text{ mcg}$$

Infusion Rate (IR) from Dose/Hr

$$\frac{\text{Dose/hour desired}}{\text{Concentration}} = \text{IR (mL/hr or gtt/min)}$$

Example: A patient is to receive 1.0 gm/hr of Amicar from a concentration of 15 gm Amicar/500 mL D$_5$W (0.03 gm/mL), so

$$\frac{1.0 \text{ gm/hr}}{15 \text{ gm/500 mL (0.03 gm/mL)}} = 33 \text{ mL/hr (gtt/min)}$$

Infusion Rate (IR) from Dose/Min

$$\frac{\text{Desired dose/min} \times 60 \text{ gtt/mL}}{\text{Concentration}} = \text{IR in mL/hr (gtt/min)}$$

Example: A patient is to receive 400 mcg/minute of dopamine from a concentration of 400 mg dopamine/500 mL D_5W (800 mcg/mL), so

$$\frac{400 \text{ mcg/min} \times 60 \text{ gtt/mL}}{800 \text{ mcg/mL}} = 30 \text{ mL/hr (gtt/min)}$$

Infusion Rate (IR) from mcg/kg/min

$$\frac{\text{Body weight in kg} \times \text{desired dose in mcg/kg/min}}{\text{Concentration in mcg/gtt}} = \text{IR (pump setting)}$$

Example: A 60-kg patient is to receive a 10-mcg/kg/min dopamine infusion from a concentration of 400 mg/500 mL D_5W (13.3 mcg/gtt), so

$$\frac{60 \text{ kg} \times 10 \text{ mcg/kg/min}}{13.3 \text{ mcg/gtt}} = \text{IR (pump setting) or 45 mL/hr (gtt/min)}$$

CLASSIFICATION OF ANTIARRHYTHMIC DRUGS

CLASS I
- Local anesthetics
- Suppress sodium ion influx
- Depress depolarization

Subclass/Name	Action
Ia Disopyramide Procainamide Quinidine	• Reduce ectopy • Suppress reentry circuits • Prolong QT interval • Increase PR interval (initially may reduce PR interval) • Widen QRS complex • May increase LVEDP • May decrease cardiac output
Ib Lidocaine Mexiletine Phenytoin Tocainide	• Reduce ectopy • Hasten repolarization • May shorten QT interval
Ic Encainide Flecainide Indecainide Lorcainide	• Slow intracardiac conduction • Prolong PR interval • Widen QRS without prolonging QT interval

CLASS II
- Beta-blockers
- Slow rate of SA node
- Slow conduction through AV node

Name	Action

Acebutolol
Atenolol
Esmolol
Metoprolol
Nadolol
Pindolol
Propranolol
Timolol
	• Reduce
	  – HR
	  – myocardial contractility
	  – myocardial O_2 demands
	• Increase
	  – PR interval
	  – bronchial constriction

CLASS III

- Act on reentry circuits
- Prolong repolarization

Name
Amiodarone
Bretylium
Sotalol

Action
- Reduce intraventricular conduction

CLASS IV

- Calcium channel blockers

Name
Diltiazem
Nifedipine
Verapamil

Action
- Reduce HR
- Increase PR interval

ACEBUTOLOL HCL (SECTRAL)

Classification: Cardioselective beta-blocker, antihypertensive,
antiarrhythmic (Type II)

Indications
Hypertension, ventricular tachydysrhythmias. **Unlabeled uses:** prophylaxis of myocardial infarction, treatment of angina, mitral valve prolapse, idiopathic hypertrophic subaortic stenosis, anxiety, tremors, thyrotoxicosis. Therapeutic effect: decreased heart rate, decreased AV conduction, decreased B/P

Contraindications
Persistent severe bradycardia, second- and third-degree heart block, cardiac failure, uncompensated congestive heart failure, pulmonary edema

Preparation/Administration†	Compatibilities	Adverse Effects	Drug Interactions
• PO administration: 400–800 mg daily, single or divided dose – not to exceed 1200 mg daily • May be administered with food or on empty stomach **Abrupt withdrawal may result in life-threatening dysrhythmias, hypertension, or myocardial ischemia.** *Sectral is dialyzable	(See drug interactions	• Bradycardia • CHF/pulmonary edema • Hypotension • Bronchospasm/ wheezing • Peripheral vasoconstriction • Hyper/hypo-glycemia • CNS changes – anxiety – depression – nervousness	• Additive myocardial depression with – verapamil – IV phenytoin – general anesthesia • Additive brady-cardia with – cardiac glycosides • Additive hypo-tension with – nitrates

- drowsiness
- dizziness

- antihypertensive
  agents
- alcohol
- Unopposed
  alpha-adrenergic
  stimulation with
  - epinephrine
- Decreased
  effectiveness with
  - thyroid
    preparations
- Prolonged
  hypoglycemia with
  - insulin

---

†Take apical pulse prior to administration; if <50 beats per minute or dysrhythmia occurs, withhold medication.

ACTIVASE® (ALTEPLASE)

Classification: Tissue plasminogen activator, thrombolytic agent

The risks of activase therapy may be increased and should be weighed against anticipated benefits under the following conditions:

- Recent (within 10 days) major surgery, such as
  - coronary artery bypass graft
  - obstetrical delivery
  - organ biopsy
  - previous puncture of noncompressible vessels (including central lines)
- Cerebrovascular disease
- GI or GU bleeding
- Recent (within 10 days) trauma (including CPR)
- Hypertension
  - systolic ≥180 mm Hg
  - diastolic ≥110 mm Hg
- High likelihood of left-heart thrombus (e.g., mitral stenosis with atrial fibrillation)
- Acute pericarditis
- Hemostatic defects, including those secondary to severe hepatic or renal disease
- Subacute bacterial endocarditis
- Significant liver dysfunction
- Pregnancy
- Diabetic hemorrhagic retinopathy or other hemorrhagic ophthalmic conditions
- Septic thrombophlebitis or occluded AV cannula at seriously infected site

- Advanced age (i.e., over 75 years old)
- Patients currently receiving oral anticoagulants (e.g., warfarin sodium)
- Any other condition where bleeding constitutes a significant hazard or would be particularly difficult to manage because of location

Indications

Acute MI (AMI) in adults for lysis of thrombi obstructing coronary arteries, reduction of infarct size, improvement of ventricular function following an MI, reduction of incidence of CHF associated with MI, reduction of motality associated with AMI, pulmonary embolism. Therapeutic effect: lysis of coronary thrombi, subsequent limitation of infarct size, lysis of life-threatening pulmonary emboli

Treatment should be initiated as soon as possible after onset of symptoms.

Actions
- Prevents death of myocardial tissue
- Fibrin-enhanced conversion of plasminogen to plasmin
- Produces limited conversion of plasminogen in the absence of fibrin
- Systemically binds to fibrin in a thrombus and converts entrapped plasminogen to plasmin
- Local fibrinolysis with limited systemic proteolysis

Contraindications

Active internal bleeding, history of cerebrovascular accident, recent (within 2 months) intracranial or intraspinal surgery/trauma, intracranial neoplasm, arteriovenous malformation or aneurysm, known bleeding diathesis, severe uncontrolled hypertension

Reconstitution/Dilution

For 100 mg vials (do not use if vacuum present)

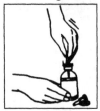

1. Insert one end of transfer device into the vial containing the diluent.

Remove the protective flip-caps from both vials. Open the package containing the transfer device by peeling back the paper label. Remove the protective cap from one end of the transfer device. Insert the exposed piercing pin of the transfer device into the vial containing the diluent. **DO NOT INVERT THE DILUENT VIAL.**

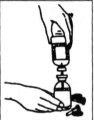

2. Holding the Activase® (Alteplase, recombinant) vial upside-down, insert the other end of the transfer device into the center of the stopper.

Remove the protective cap from the other end of the transfer device and insert into the vial containing the Activase® lyophilized powder.

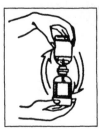

3. Invert the vials.

Invert the vials so that the diluent vial is on top and the Activase® vial is upright on the bottom. This permits all the diluent to flow freely into the Activase® vial. Because there is no vacuum present, the diluent will run smoothly and little or no foaming will occur.

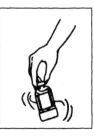

4. Inspect the solution.

Allow the entire contents of the vial to run into the Activase® vial (approximately 0.5 cc of diluent will remain in the diluent vial). Remove the empty vial and transfer device as one unit and safely discard. Gently swirl the vial and examine the contents. Reconstituted preparation results in a transparent pale yellow to colorless solution. If solution is discolored or particulate matter is seen, do not use.

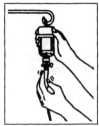

5. Hang the 100 mg vial for direct infusion and prime the tubing.

The Activase® vial has a plastic molded cap with a loop attached to the bottom so that it can be hung for direct infusion. If you prefer, the contents of the vial can be transferred to an IV bag.

Reconstitution and Dilution for 100 mg Vial (Figures 8.1 to 8.5) reprinted with permission from Genentech, Inc. (South San Francisco, CA), May 1992.

Special Considerations
- IV use only
- In case of serious bleeding not controlled by local pressure, infusion of Activase® and heparin should be terminated immediately; heparin may be reversed by protamine; clotting factors may be replaced by fresh frozen plasma or cryoprecipitate
- Obtaining lab samples (if A-line is unavailable):
  - use previously established IV site (before initiation of Activase® at this site)
  - discard first 3–5 mL of blood obtained
  - continue to obtain blood for lab sample

Compatibilities
- As a general guideline, no other medication should be added to Activase® or in the line being used for Activase®
- If the clinical situation warrants, the following drugs are acceptable for piggybacking (simultaneous administration) through the same tubing:
  - lidocaine
  - propranolol HCl
  - metoprolol tartrate

Incompatibilities with Activase® solutions
  - heparin (lowers Alteplase activity)
  - morphine (activity is reduced by Alteplase)

Adverse Effects
- Bleeding
  - active internal bleeding involving
    - GI tract
    - GU tract
    - cardiac catheterization site
    - intracranial sites
  - surface or superficial bleeding, observed mainly at disturbed or invaded sites
    - arterial punctures
    - venous cutdowns
    - sites of recent surgical intervention
- Hypersensitivity reactions, such as
  - urticaria
  - nausea
  - vomiting
  - hypotension
  - laryngeal edema
  - fever

Drug Interactions
- Drugs that alter platelet function may increase the risk of bleeding if administered prior to, during, or after Activase® therapy, i.e.,
  - acetylsalicylic acid (aspirin)
  - dipyridamole (Persantin)

Special Considerations
- During infusion of Activase®, if arterial/venipuncture is necessary, select a vessel accessible to manual compression; pressure should be applied for 30 min
  - avoid IM injections

Incompatibilities
- dopamine (reduces Alteplase activity and can result in particulate formation)
- dobutamine (can result in precipitate formation)
- Dilution of Alteplase beyond 0.5 mg/mL is not recommended (may result in precipitation of Alteplase protein)

Adverse Effects
- Reperfusion dysrhythmias, such as
  - sinus bradycardia
  - accelerated idioventricular rhythm
  - PVCs
  - ventricular tachycardia
- Ecchymosis and/or inflammation at IV site

*Although not directly attributable to Alteplase therapy, some adverse reactions have been reported (i.e., pulmonary edema, heart failure, recurrent ischemia, reinfarction, myocardial rupture, mitral regurgitation, pericardial effusion, pericarditis, cardiac tamponade, cardiac arrest, venous thrombosis/embolism, and electromechanical dissociation)

Dosage/Administration—Acute Myocardial Infarction (3-hr infusion)

Administer Activase® as soon as possible after the onset of symptoms.

- Administer by IV infusion only
- Recommended dose *not* to exceed 100 mg
- Initial dose is 6–10 mg IV push over first 1–2 min
- Follow with 50 mg over first hour as continuous infusion
- Follow with 20 mg over second hour as continuous infusion
- Follow with 20 mg over third hour as continuous infusion
    a. The **bolus dose** may be prepared in one of the following ways:
        1. By removing 6–10 mL from the vial of reconstituted (1 mg/mL) Activase® using a syringe and needle. If this method is used with the 20 mg or 50 mg vials, the syringe should not be primed with air and the needle should be inserted into the Activase® vial stopper. If the 100 mg vial is used, the needle should be inserted away from the puncture mark made by the transfer device.
        2. By removing 6–10 mL from a port (second injection site) on the infusion line after the infusion set is primed.
        3. By programming an infusion pump to deliver a 6–10 mL (1 mg/mL) bolus at the initiation of the infusion.
    b. The remainder of the Activase® dose may be administered as follows:
        1. ***20 mg, 50 mg vials***—administer using either a polyvinyl chloride bag or glass vial infusion set.
        2. ***100 mg vials***—insert the spike end of an infusion set through the same puncture site created by the transfer device in the stopper of the vial of reconstituted Activase®. Hang the Activase® vial from the plastic-molded capping attached to the bottom of the vial. (See Figures 8.1–8.5, page 318)
- When IV bag is empty, add 25 mL of nonbacteriostatic IV solution (0.9% NaCl or D_5W) and allow to infuse at previously set rate.
- For patients weighing less than 65 kg, administer dose of 1.25 mg/kg: 60% of total dose (of which 6%–10% administered as bolus) over first hour, 20% over second hour, and 20% over the third hour. (See chart on page 322.)

Dosing Information for AMI: 3-hr regimen
3-hr dose: 100 mg Activase® over 3 hrs
Weight-adjusted dose for patients <65 kg: 1.25 mg/ kg Activase® over 3 hrs

Dose by Weight for Patients < 65 kg:

Weight (kg)	Total dose (mg)
64	80
60	75
55	69
50	63
45	56
40	50

Dosage Schedule for AMI: 3-hr regimen

Lytic dose	First hour	60% of total dose (of which 6%–10% is administered as bolus)
Maintenance dose	Second hour	20% of total dose
	Third hour	20% of total dose

The most effective and least complicated method of administering IV drugs is with tubing that delivers 60 gtts/cc.

Dosing Information for AMI, 3-hr regimen for patients <65 kg: 1.25 mg/kg reprinted with permission from Genentech, Inc. (South San Francisco, CA), March 1995.

Dosage/Administration—Acute Myocardial Infarction (Accelerated Regimen)

- Administer by IV infusion only
- Based on patient weight, not to exceed 100 mg
- Patients weighing >67 kg = >147.5 lb
  - administer 15 mg (15 mL) bolus
  - administer 50 mg over next 30 min
  - administer 35 mg over next 60 min
  * total dose = 100 mg/90 min
- Patients weighing ≤67 kg (≤147.5 lb)
  - administer 15 mg (15 mL) bolus
  - administer 0.75 mg/kg over next 30 min *(not to exceed 50 mg)*
  - administer 0.50 mg/kg over next 60 min *(not to exceed 35 mg)*
  * total dose <100 mg/90 min—refer to chart on p. 324
  a. The **bolus dose** may be prepared in one of the following ways:
    1. Remove 15 mL from the vial of reconstituted Activase® (1 mg/mL) using a syringe and needle. With 20 mg or 50 mg vials, *do not* prime the syringe with air. The needle should be inserted into the Activase® vial stopper. If using the 100 mg vial, the needle should be inserted away from the puncture mark made by the transfer device.
    2. Remove 15 mg from a port on the infusion line (second injection site) after the infusion tubing is primed.
    3. Program an infusion pump to deliver a 15 mL (1 mg/mL) bolus at initiation of infusion.
  b. The remainder of the Activase® dose may be administered as per the 3-hr infusion regimen (b), page 321.

Accelerated Regimen for Patients—Dose by Weight for Patients ≤67 kg (≤147.5 lb)*

Weight (kg)	Weight (lb)	Total dose (mg)	Bolus dose (mg)	Next 30 min			Next 60 min		
				Infusion dose (mg)	Infusion rate (mL/h)	Volume to be infused (mL)	Infusion dose (mg)	Infusion rate (mL/h)	Volume to be infused (mL)
41	90	66.5	15	31	62	31	20.5	20.5	20.5
42	92.5	67.5	15	31.5	63	31.5	21	21	21
43	94.5	68.5	15	32	64	32	21.5	21.5	21.5
44	97	70	15	33	66	33	22	22	22
45	99	71.5	15	34	68	34	22.5	22.5	22.5
46	101	72.5	15	34.5	69	34.5	23	23	23
47	103.5	73.5	15	35	70	35	23.5	23.5	23.5
48	105.5	75	15	36	72	36	24	24	24
49	108	76.5	15	37	74	37	24.5	24.5	24.5
50	110	77.5	15	37.5	75	37.5	25	25	25
51	112	78.5	15	38	76	38	25.5	25.5	25.5
52	114.5	80	15	39	78	39	26	26	26
53	116.5	81.5	15	40	80	40	26.5	26.5	26.5
54	119	82.5	15	40.5	81	40.5	27	27	27
55	121	83.5	15	41	82	41	27.5	27.5	27.5
56	123	85	15	42	84	42	28	28	28
57	125.5	86.5	15	43	86	43	28.5	28.5	28.5
58	127.5	87.5	15	43.5	87	43.5	29	29	29
59	130	88.5	15	44	88	44	29.5	29.5	29.5

60	132	90	15	45	90	45	30	30	30
61	134	91.5	15	46	92	46	30.5	30.5	30.5
62	136.5	92.5	15	46.5	93	46.5	31	31	31
63	138.5	93.5	15	47	94	47	31.5	31.5	31.5
64	141	95	15	48	96	48	32	32	32
65	143	96.5	15	49	98	49	32.5	32.5	32.5
66	145	97.5	15	49.5	99	49.5	33	33	33
67	147.5	98.5	15	50	100	50	33.5	33.5	33.5

*Activase® solution of 1 mg/mL

Reprinted with permission from Genentech, Inc. (460 Point San Bruno Blvd, San Francisco, CA 94080-4990), March 1995.

Dosage/Administration—Pulmonary Embolism
- The recommended dose is 100 mg administered by IV infusion over 2 hr
- Heparin therapy should be instituted or reinstituted near the end of or immediately following the Activase® infusion when the partial thromboplastin time or thrombin time returns to twice normal or less
- The dose may be administered using the instructions described in Dosage/Administration for Myocardial Infarction—3 hr regimen (b), page 321

ACTIVASE TREATMENT ALGORITHM

PRETREATMENT INTERVENTION

History Assessment		Consent

LAB

EKG	PT, PTT	Fibrinogen level	CBC with Platelets	CPK, CPK-MB	SMA-20	Type and Screen 2-4 units PRBCs	ABC

PATIENT PREPARATION

Establish 2-3 IV sites	No central line	Lidocaine 100 mg IV bolus followed by 2 mg/min	IV NTG may be indicated to relieve chest pain or control blood pressure	Atropine and Isuprel available

No foley

Temporary external pacemaker available

DRUG PREPARATION

Reconstitute Activase	→	In diluent supplied by manufacturer	→	Following reconstitution can be diluted 1:2	→	Normal Diluent: Saline or D₅W

*Refer to available information on how the drug is supplied

Figure 8.6   Activase Treatment Algorithm

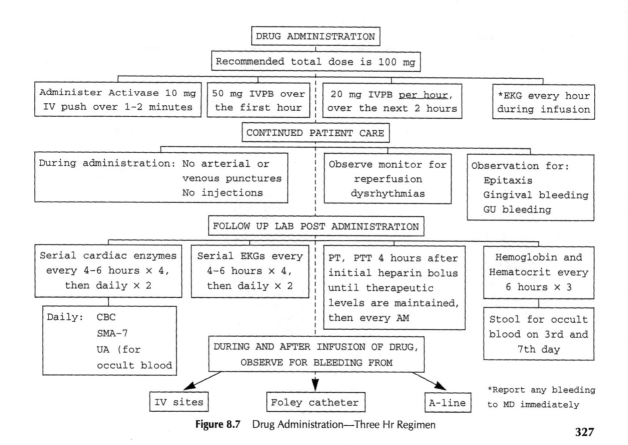

DRUG ADMINISTRATION

Recommended total dose is 100 mg

| Administer Activase 10 mg IV push over 1-2 minutes | 50 mg IVPB over the first hour | 20 mg IVPB per hour, over the next 2 hours | *EKG every hour during infusion |

CONTINUED PATIENT CARE

| During administration: No arterial or venous punctures No injections | Observe monitor for reperfusion dysrhythmias | Observation for: Epitaxis Gingival bleeding GU bleeding |

FOLLOW UP LAB POST ADMINISTRATION

| Serial cardiac enzymes every 4-6 hours × 4, then daily × 2 | Serial EKGs every 4-6 hours × 4, then daily × 2 | PT, PTT 4 hours after initial heparin bolus until therapeutic levels are maintained, then every AM | Hemoglobin and Hematocrit every 6 hours × 3 |

Daily: CBC
        SMA-7
        UA (for
        occult blood

Stool for occult blood on 3rd and 7th day

DURING AND AFTER INFUSION OF DRUG, OBSERVE FOR BLEEDING FROM

IV sites   Foley catheter   A-line

*Report any bleeding to MD immediately

Figure 8.7   Drug Administration—Three Hr Regimen

327

ADENOSINE (ADENOCARD)

Classification: Antiarrhythmic, nucleoside

Indications
Initial conversion of PSVT. Therapeutic effect: restoration of normal sinus rhythm

Contraindications
Sick sinus syndrome, second- or third-degree AV block (except in patients with functioning artificial pacemaker), sensitivity to adenosine

Preparation/Administration	Compatibilities	Adverse Effects[†]	Drug Interactions

• IV bolus: 6 mg over 2 sec; follow with rapid saline flush
  – repeat, if indicated, in 1–2 min with 12 mg over 2 sec
  – may repeat 12 mg bolus
 	
Single doses >12 mg are not recommended
	• NaCl 0.9%	• Varying degrees of heart block
		• Nonsustained ventricular tachycardia
		• PVCs
		• PACs
		• Sinus tachycardia
		• Sinus bradycardia
		• Chest pain
		• Chest pressure
		• Palpitations
		• Hypotension
			• Inhibits adenosine uptake
			  – dipyridamole
			  – carbamazepine
			  – theophyllin
			  – caffeine

- Dyspnea, shortness of breath
- Hyperventilation
- Facial flushing
- Nausea
- Headache, dizziness
- Lightheadedness
- Apprehension
- Metallic taste
- Tightness in throat

---

†The half-life of adenosine is less than 10 sec. Adverse effects are usually self-limiting. Treatment of prolonged adverse effects should be individualized to the specific effect.

AMINOPHYLLINE (AMINOPHYLLIN, PHYLLOCONTIN)

Classification: Spasmolytic, bronchodilator

Indications
Bronchospasm, status asthmaticus, CHF, Cheyne–Stokes respirations, cardiac dyspnea, exertional dyspnea with emphysema. Therapeutic effect: bronchodilation

Contraindications
Known hypersensitivity to xanthine or ethylenediamine, hyperthyroidism, uncontrolled dysrhythmias

Preparation/Administration
- Give slowly IV (undiluted or diluted in compatible solution)
- Rate: not to exceed 25 mg/min
- Loading dose: 6 mg/kg
- Maintenance dose: 0.1–1.0 mg/kg/hr

Therapeutic drug levels should be monitored. The therapeutic range is 10–20 mcg/mL.

Utilize infusion pump to ensure accurate dosage.

Compatibilities
- D_5W
- D_5/0.2% NaCl
  0.45% NaCl
  0.9% NaCl
- D_5 Ringer's
- D_5 lactated Ringer's
- Ringer's
- Lactated Ringer's
- NaCl 0.45%
  0.9%
- Amrinone (INOCOR)
- Bretylium
- Calcium gluconate
- Dexamethasone (Decadron)
- Dopamine
- Heparin

Adverse Effects (Dose dependent)
- Respiratory arrest
- Tachycardia
- Seizure
- Hypotension
- Palpitations/angina
- Anxiety
- Restlessness
- Dizziness
- Insomnia
- Headache
- Lightheadedness

Drug Interactions
- Decreases the therapeutic effect of lithium
- May potentiate the toxic effects of cardiac glycosides
- Synergistic toxicity with ephedrine and other sympathomimetics
- May enhance effects of oral anti-coagulants
  – increased plasma prothrombin and factor V

- Lidocaine
- Nitroglycerin
- Potassium chloride
- Sodium bicarbonate
- Verapamil

Theophyllin may cause or worsen dysrhythmias. Any significant change in rate and/or rhythm warrants monitoring and appropriate treatment.

Drug half-life
- decreased
  - smokers
  - alcoholics
  - marijuana smokers
  - rifampin
  - phenobarbital
- increased
  - renal, hepatic, or cardiac failure
  - respiratory infection
  - COPD

- Decreased hepatic clearance related to cimetidine, high-dose allopurinol, propranolol, erythromycin, oral contraceptives, amiodarone

AMIODARONE (CORDARONE)

Classification: Antiarrhythmic (Class III), adrenergic blocker

Indications

Refractory ventricular or supraventricular dysrhythmias, Wolff–Parkinson–White (WPW) syndrome, atrial fibrillation/flutter. Therapeutic effect: suppression of ventricular dysrhythmias

Contraindications

Severe sinus node dysfunction, second- and third-degree AV block, bradycardia (unless a functioning artificial pacemaker is in place)

Preparation/Administration	**Compatibilities**	**Adverse Effects**	**Drug Interactions**

• PO (adult), loading dose: 800–1600 mg/daily for 1–3 wks or until therapeutic response is evident
  – maintenance dose: 600–800 mg/daily for about 4 wks, then further reduced to lowest effective dose, usually 400 mg/daily
	(See Drug Interactions)	• CHF
		• Hypotension
		• Bradycardia
		• Peripheral vasodilation
		• Headache
		• Depression
		• Insomnia
		• Tremor
		• Anorexia
		• Abdominal pain
			• Digoxin (decrease dose by 50%)
			• Increases
			  – blood levels of phenytoin
			  – activity of warfarin
			  – blood levels of flecainide
			• Beta-blockers/calcium channel blockers
			  – increased risk of dysrhythmias

Effects after discontinuation of the drug may last for weeks.

Therapeutic drug levels should be monitored.

Therapeutic range:
0.5–2.5 mcg/mL.

**Amiodarone is a highly
toxic drug. The lowest
effective dose should be
utilized.**

AMIODARONE (CORDARONE) INTRAVENOUS

Classification: Antiarrhythmic (Class III)[†]

Indications**
Initiation of treatment, prophylaxis of frequently recurring ventricular fibrillation and hemodynamically unstable ventricular tachycardia, refractory to other therapy. VT/VF for patients unable to take oral medication. *During or after treatment with Cordarone IV, patients must be transferred to oral Cordarone.*
Therapeutic effect: reduces frequency of arrhythmic events

Contraindications
Cardiogenic shock, marked sinus bradycardia, second- or third-degree AV block in the absence of a functioning pacemaker, known hypersensitivity to any of the components of Cordarone IV

[†]Although it is a Class III, it possesses electrophysiologic characteristics of all four classes.

**This drug should be administered by physicians experienced in the treatment of life-threatening arrhythmias, thoroughly familiar with the risks and benefits of Cordarone therapy and only by those who have access to adequate monitoring capabilities.

Preparation/Administration
- A CVC should be utilized for concentrations greater than 2 mg/mL
- Concentrations greater than 3 mg/mL demonstrate a high incidence of peripheral vein phlebitis
- An in-line filter is recommended
- Transition to oral therapy should be initiated at the earliest possible time
- When administering Cordarone, a volumetric pump must be used

Loading Infusion	**Compatibilities**	**Adverse Effects**	**Drug Interactions**

• *First* rapid
  – concentration: 1.5 mg/mL (150 mg in 100 mL D$_5$W)
  – rate: 15 mg/min (100 mL over **first** 10 min)
  – container: PVC or glass
	• D$_5$W
	Incompatibilities
	• Aminophyllin
	• Cefamandole nafate
	• Cefazolin sodium
	• Heparin
	• Mezlocillin sodium
	• Sodium bicarbonate
		• Hypotension
		• Asystole/cardiac arrest/pulseless electrical activity (EMD)
		• VT
		• Cardiogenic shock
		• CHF
		• Bradycardia
		• AV block
		• Abnormalities of liver function tests
			• Warfarin
			  – increased prothrombin time
			• Digoxin, quinidine
			  – increased serum concentration
			• Procainamide
			  – increased serum concentration and NAPA concentration
			• Disopyramide
			  – QT prolongation
			• Fentanyl
			  – hypotension
			  – bradycardia
			  – decreased cardiac output

- **Followed** by slow
  - concentration: 1.8 mg/mL (900 mg in 500 mL D$_5$W)
  - rate: 1 mg/min (33.3 mL/hr) over the next 6 hr)
  - container: glass or polyolefin

- Flecainide
  - increases plasma concentration (reduce dose)
- Lidocaine with IV Cordarone
  - seizures
- Cyclosporine
  - persistently elevated plasma concentrations
  - elevated creatinine
- Cholestyramine
  - decreased serum level of Cordarone
- Cimetidine
  - increases serum Cordarone level
- Phenytoin
  - decreases serum Cordarone level
- Beta-blockers
  - increased risk of hypotension and bradycardia

Maintenance Infusion

- *Over remaining 18 hr— 540 mg*
  - concentration: 1.8 mg/mL
  - rate: reduce **to 0.5 mg/min** (16.6 mL/hr)
  - container: glass or polyolefin
- *After first 24 hr,* maintenance infusion at a rate of 0.5 mg/min (720 mg/24 hr) should be continued, maintaining a concentration of 1–6 mg/mL

Supplemental Infusion

- For management of breakthrough episodes of life-threatening VT or VF. *Alternatively,* the rate of maintenance infusion may be increased
  - concentration: 1.5 mg/mL (150 mg in 100 mL D_5W)
  - rate: 15 mg/min (100 mL over 10 min)
  - container: PVC or glass
- To protect from light, store ampules in cartons until ready for use
- Discard prepared solutions after 24 hr

Drug Interactions (*cont.*)

- Calcium channel blockers
  - inhibited AV conduction
  - decreased myocardial contractility
  - hypotension
- Calan or diltiazem
  - increases risk of AV block

AMRINONE (INOCOR)

Classification: Inotropic agent

Indications
CHF unresponsive to conventional therapy. Therapeutic effect: suppression of ventricular dysrhythmias

Contraindications
Patients with aortic or pulmonic valvular disease. **Note:** Use *cautiously* in patients with hypertropic subaortic stenosis, acute myocardial infarction

Preparation/Administration
- IV: bolus of 0.75 mg/kg over 2–3 min
  - maintenance: 5–10 mcg/kg/min
- Total daily dose *not to exceed* 10 mg/kg

Compatibilities
- Y-site compatibility
  - aminophyllin
  - atropine
  - bretylium
  - calcium chloride
  - cimetidine
  - dobutamine
  - dopamine
  - epinephrine
  - isoproterenol
  - lidocaine
  - nitroglycerine
  - nitroprusside
  - norepinephrine
  - phenylephrine
  - potassium chloride
  - procainamide
  - verapamil

Adverse Effects
- Cardiac dysrhythmias
- Hypotension
- Chest pain
- Hypersensitivity
- Nausea/vomiting
- Cramps
- Liver enzyme elevation

Drug Interactions
- Increased inotropic effects with
  - cardiac glycosides
- Hypotension exaggerated by
  - disopyramide

Loading Dose Determination[†]

Patient weight (kg)	30	40	50	60	70	80	90	100	110	120
mL of undiluted INOCOR injection	4.5	6.0	7.5	9.0	10.5	12.0	13.5	15.0	16.5	18.0

IV Infusion Rate (mL/hr) Chart[‡]

Patient weight (kg)	30	40	50	60	70	80	90	100	110	120
Dosage (mcg/kg/min)										
5.0	4	5	6	7	8	10	11	12	13	14
7.5	5	7	9	11	13	14	16	18	20	22
10.0	7	10	12	14	17	19	22	24	26	29

[†]0.75 mg/kg (undiluted)

[‡]Using 2.5 mg/mL infusion concentration

Example: A 70-kg patient would require a loading dose of 10.5 mL of undiluted INOCOR. If the physician selects a dose of 7.5 µg/kg/min for the infusion, the flow rate would be 13 mL/hr for the 2.5 mg/mL concentration of INOCOR.

Dilution: To prepare the 2.5 mg/mL concentration recommended for infusion, mix INOCOR with an equal volume of diluent. For example, mix three 20-mL ampuls of INOCOR (3 × 20 mL = 60 mL) with 60 mL of diluent for a total volume of 120 mL of the final 2.5-mg/mL solution of INOCOR.

Do not dilute amrinone with solutions containing dextrose; diluted amrinone may be piggybacked into an established dextrose infusion.

The most effective and least complicated method of administering IV drugs is with tubing that delivers 60 gtts/cc.

When administering INOCOR, adhere strictly to the charts prepared by the manufacturer. **Refer to full package insert for full prescribing information.**

INOCOR Loading Dose Determination, Infusion Rate Chart, and examples reprinted with permission from Sanofi Winthrop Pharmaceuticals (New York), November 1993 product information.

ANISTREPLASE (EMINASE)

Classification: Thrombolytic agent

The risks of Eminase therapy may be increased and should be weighed against anticipated benefits under the following conditions:

- Recent (within 10 days) major surgery, such as
  - coronary artery bypass graft
  - obstetrical delivery
  - organ biopsy
  - previous puncture of noncompressible vessels (including central lines)
- Cerebrovascular disease
- Recent (within 10 days) GI or GU bleeding
- Recent (within 10 days) trauma (including CPR)
- Hypertension
  - systolic ≥180 mm Hg
  - diastolic ≥110 mm Hg
- High likelihood of left-heart thrombus (e.g., mitral stenosis with atrial fibrillation)
- Subacute bacterial endocarditis
- Aute pericarditis
- Hemostatic defects, including those secondary to severe hepatic or renal disease
- Pregnancy
- Advanced age (i.e., over 75 years old); use of Eminase in patients over 75 years old has not been adequately studied
- Diabetic hemorrhagic retinopathy or other hemorrhagic ophthalmic conditions
- Septic thrombophlebitis or occluded AV cannula at seriously infected site

- Patients currently receiving oral anticoagulants (e.g., warfarin sodium)
- Any other condition where bleeding constitutes a significant hazard or would be particularly difficult to manage because of location

Indications
Acute myocardial infarction, lysis of thrombi obstructing coronary arteries, reduction of infarct size, improvement of ventricular function and reduction of mortality associated with AMI. **TREATMENT SHOULD BE INITIATED AS SOON AS POSSIBLE AFTER ONSET OF SYMPTOMS.** Therapeutic effect: lysis of thrombi in coronary arteries with preservation of ventricular function

Actions
Conversion of plasminogen to plasmin with subsequent fibrinolysis

Contraindications
Active internal bleeding, history of CVA, recent (within 2 months) intracranial or intraspinal surgery or trauma, intracranial neoplasm, aneurysm or AV malformation, severe uncontrolled hypertension, known bleeding diathesis.

Eminase should not be administered to patients having experienced allergic reactions to either Eminase or Streptokinase.

Pretreatment Labs
Hematocrit, hemoglobin, platelet count, PT/PTT, bleeding time, APTT, fibrinogen degradation products, type and match, have blood available

Reconstitution

- The reconstituted solution should not be further diluted before administration or added to any infusion fluids. No other medications should be added to the vial or syringe containing Eminase
- To the vial of Eminase powder, slowly add 5 mL of sterile water for injection, USP. **Direct stream of fluid against the side of the vial to minimize foaming of the solution.**
- Gently roll the vial, mixing the fluid with the dry powder—**do not shake**
- The reconstituted preparation is colorless to pale yellow and is transparent; visually inspect the finished product for particulate matter or discoloration
- Withdraw the entire contents of the vial
- **Recommended dose:** 30 units of Eminase by IV injection over 2–5 min
- Discard Eminase not administered within 30 min of recon-

Adverse Effects

- Severe hypotension
- Bleeding
- Dysrhythmias
- Bronchospasm
- Allergic reactions

Drug Interactions

- Interactions with other cardio-active drugs has not been studied
- Drugs that alter platelet function (aspirin/dipyridamole) may increase bleeding risk

ATENOLOL (TENORMIN)

Classification: Antihypertensive, antianginal, beta-adrenergic blocker

Indications
Treatment of mild to moderate hypertension, angina pectoris, prevention/management of MI. **Unlabeled uses:** management of dysrhythmias, mitral valve prolapse, vascular headache, hypertropic cardiomyopathy, tremors, thyrotoxicosis, pheochromocytoma. Therapeutic effect: decreased heart rate, decreased B/P, prevention of myocardial infarction

Contraindications
Patients with cardiac failure, cardiogenic shock, second- or third-degree AV block, sinus bradycardia, CHF, pulmonary edema; may mask symptoms of thyrotoxicosis, diabetes; dosage reduction required in renal impairment

Preparation/Administration
- Hypertension: 50–100 mg PO daily
- Angina: 50–200 mg PO daily
- Myocardial infarction
  - initial 5 mg IV over 5 min
  - can be followed by another 5 mg IV 10 min later

Compatibilities
- D_5W
- D_5 0.9% NaCl
- NaCl 0.9%

These admixtures are stable for 48 hr

Adverse Effects
- Bronchospasm/wheezing
- Pulmonary edema
- CHF
- Hypotension
- Bradycardia

Drug Interactions
- Additive myocardial depression with
  - general anesthesia
  - dilantin (IV)
  - verapamil
- Increased bradycardia with
  - cardiac glycosides
- Increased hypotension with
  - antihypertensive agents
  - nitrates

Preparation/Administration

– for patients who tolerate the 10-mg dose (IV), start 50-mg PO, 10 min after the last IV dose; follow with 50 mg (PO) in 12 hr. Therefore 100 mg (PO) daily or in 2 divided doses (50 mg BID)

– may be given for 6–9 days, PO, or until discharged from hospital

Abrupt withdrawal may precipitate life-threatening dysrhythmias, hypertension, or myocardial ischemia

*Moderately dialyzable (20%–50%)

Drug Interactions

- Decreased effectiveness with
  – thyroid supplements
- Alpha-adrenergic stimulation increased with
  – epinephrine
- Decreased bronchodilation with
  – theophyllin

ATROPINE

Classification: Antiarrhythmic, parasympatholytic

Indications
Bradycardia, bradydysrhythmias, antispasmodic, antidote for organophosphate pesticide poisoning. Therapeutic effect: increases heart rate, bronchodilation, decreases GI and respiratory secretions, spasmolytic action on the biliary and genitourinary tract

Contraindications
Narrow-angle glaucoma, tachycardia, thyrotoxicosis, hypersensitivity to belladonna alkaloids, acute hemorrhage

Preparation/Administration
- IV bolus: 0.5–1.0 mg
  - repeat in 5 min
  - do not exceed 2 mg

Doses lower than 0.5 mg can cause bradycardia

Compatibilities
- Dextrose solutions
- Saline solutions
- Lactated Ringer's
- Amrinone
- Dobutamine
- Heparin
- Hydrocortisone
- Meperidine
- Morphine
- Potassium chloride
- Procainamide
- Ranitidine
- Verapamil

Incompatibilities
- Norepinephrine
- Sodium bicarbonate

Adverse Effects
- Cardiac dysrhythmias
- Impaired GI motility
- Urinary hesitancy, retention
- Palpitations
- Drowsiness
- Confusion
- Blurred vision
- Constipation

Drug Interactions
- Additive anticholinergic effect
  - antihistamines
  - tricyclic antidepressants
  - quinidine
  - disopyramide
  - phenothiazines

345

BRETYLIUM TOSYLATE (BRETYLOL, BRETYLATE)

Classification: Antiarrhythmic (Class III), beta-blocker

Indications
Prophylaxis and treatment of ventricular dysrhythmia unresponsive to lidocaine. Therapeutic effect: suppression of ventricular tachycardia/fibrillation

Contraindications
Digitalis-induced arrhythmias, use with caution if cardiac output impaired

Preparation/Administration	Compatibilities	Adverse Effects	Drug Interactions
• IV bolus: 5 mg/kg rapid injection – repeat in 15 min, 10 mg/kg – total dose not to exceed 30 mg/kg • IV maintenance: 1–2 mg/min **Use this drug only in a monitored situation with emergency equipment at hand.** **Dosage should be gradually reduced and discontinued over 3–5 days with close cardiac monitoring.**	• D_5W • D_5/0.45% NaCl 0.9% NaCl • D_5 lactated Ringer's • Lactated Ringer's • NaCl 0.9% • Sodium lactate ⅙ M • Aminophyllin • Amrinone lactate • Calcium chloride • Digoxin • Dopamine • Esmolol • Insulin • Isuprel • Lidocaine • Quinidine gluconate • Sodium bicarbonate • Verapamil	• Hypotension (severe postural and supine) • Bradycardia, angina • Dyspnea • Renal dysfunction • Syncopy • Pulmonary hypertension	• Cardiac glycosides – increased toxicity of these drugs • Lidocaine, procainamide, propranolol, and quinidine – neutralizes inotropic effect – potentiates hypotension • Catecholamine effect is enhanced by bretylium

IV Push Dosage Chart[†]

Patient Weight (lb)	99	110	121	132	143	154	165	176	187	198	209	220
(kg)	45	50	55	60	65	70	75	80	85	90	95	100
Dosage (mg/kg)												
5	4.5	5	5.5	6	6.5	7	7.5	8	8.5	9	9.5	10
6	5.5	6	6.6	7.2	7.8	8.4	9	9.6	10.2	10.8	11.4	12
7	6.3	7	7.7	8.4	9.1	9.8	10.5	11.2	11.9	12.6	13.3	14
8	7.2	8	8.8	9.6	10.4	11.2	12	12.8	13.6	14.4	15.2	16
9	8.1	9	9.9	10.8	11.7	12.6	13.5	14.4	15.3	16.2	17.1	18
10	9	10	11	12	13	14	15	16	17	18	19	20

Dosage/Flow-Rate Chart[‡]

Drug Dilution Concentration

Dosage (mg)	500 mg/50 mL (10 mg/mL)	500 mg/100 mL (5 mg/mL)	500 mg/250 mL (2 mg/mL)	500 mg/500 mL (1 mg/mL)
1	6	12	30	60
2	12	24	60	120
3	18	36	90	—
4	24	48	120	—

[†]Milliliters of undiluted 50 mg/mL solution to administer by IV push.

[‡]To infuse in microdrops/minute or milliliters/hour.

The most effective and least complicated method of administering IV drugs is with tubing that delivers 60 gtts/cc.

CALCIUM CHLORIDE/CALCIUM GLUCONATE

Classification: Electrolyte

Indications
Cardiac resuscitation (inotropic effect), emergency treatment of hypoglycemia, hypermagnesemia, hypocalcemia, cardiac disturbances of hyperkalemia, cardiac resuscitation when epinephrine fails to improve myocardial contraction. Therapeutic effect: replacement of calcium in deficiency states

Contraindications
Hypercalcemia, ventricular fibrillation during cardiac resuscitation, in patient with risk of digitalis toxicity, cardiac or renal disease; *may precipitate cardiac arrest*

Preparation/Administration	Compatibilities	Adverse Effects	Drug Interactions

• Emergency treatment of hypocalcemia
  – IV: 7–14 mEq
• Hypocalcemic tetany
  – IV: 4.5–16 mEq, repeat until symptoms are controlled
	• Bretylium
	• Physically compatible with
	  – digoxin
	  – isuprel
	  – lidocaine
	  – norepinephrine
	  – potassium chloride
	  – verapamil
		• Cardiac arrest
		• Cardiac dysrhythmias
		• Bradycardia
		• Hypotension
		• Hypercalcemia
		• May produce vasospasm in coronary and cerebral arteries
			• Administer cautiously to the digitalized patient
			• May antagonize effects of verapamil
			• Inactivates tetracycline antibiotics

Incompatibilities
- Magnesium sulfate
- *Calcium salts precipitate when added to*
  - carbonates
  - bicarbonates
  - phosphates
  - sulfates
  - tartrates

CAPTOPRIL (CAPOTEN)

Classification: Antihypertensive, renin–angiotensin antagonist

Indications
Chronic hypertension (usually used with a thiazide diuretic), CHF (usually used with digitalis and diuretic therapy). Therapeutic effect: lowers B/P in hypertensive patients, decreases preload/afterload in patients with CHF

Contraindications
Renal impairment, collagen vascular disease, hypersensitivity to this drug, or any other ACE inhibitor. **Note:** Use cautiously with aortic stenosis, cardiac/cerebral vascular insufficiency, surgery/anesthesia, and pregnancy (may result in malformation of fetus); use **extreme caution** with family history of hereditary angioedema

Preparation/Administration	Compatibilities	Adverse Effects	Drug Interactions

• For hypertension: (initial dose) 25 mg PO, BID, or TID
  – at intervals of 1–2 wks, dose may be increased to 50 mg BID or TID
  – dose exceeding 150 mg/daily is not usually required; if B/P control is not achieved, the addition of a thiazide diuretic should be considered
	(See Drug Interactions)	• Hypotension
		• Tachycardia
		• Angina
		• Hyperkalemia
		• Angioedema
			• Potentiated by
			  – other anti-hypertensives
			  – phenothiazines
			  – alcohol
			  – vasodilators
			• Hyperkalemia results from use of
			  – potassium supplements
			  – potassium sparing diuretics
			• Antihypertensive response inhibited by NSAIDS

Preparation/Administration

- For CHF: (initial dose)
  6.25–25 mg PO, TID
  - maintenance dose: up
    to 50 mg TID
  - *maximum dose:* 450
    mg/day

* *SHOULD BE TAKEN ONE
  HOUR BEFORE MEALS*

**Prior to starting therapy,
carefully monitor clinical
status related to previous
antihypertensive
treatment, fluid and
sodium restriction**

* Moderately dialyzable
  (20%–50%)

Drug Interactions

- Enhances activity of
  - digoxin
  - lithium
- Absorption inhibited
  by antacids
- Elimination inhibited
  by probenecid
  (increases captopril
  level)
- Hypersensitivity may
  be increased by
  allopurinol
- May increase insulin
  sensitivity

DIAZOXIDE (HYPERSTAT)

Classification: Antihypertensive, vasodilator, hyperglycemic

Indications
Emergency treatment of malignant hypertension, treatment of hypoglycemia associated with hyperinsulinism. Therapeutic effect: lowering of B/P, increased blood glucose. Hyperstat IV injection is ineffective against hypertension due to pheochromocytoma

Contraindications
Compensatory hypertension associated with arteriovenous shunt, aortic coarctation, hypersensitivity to diazoxide, other thiazides, or sulfonamide-derived drugs. **Note:** Use cautiously in diabetics, uremia, cardiovascular disease, pregnancy, and lactation

Preparation/Administration
- Hypertension
  - IV (adults): 1–3 mg/kg, undiluted, every 5–15 min
  - maximum dose 150 mg in a single dose
  - with the patient recumbent, the dose should be administered in 30 sec or less
  - should be given only in peripheral vein

*Do not administer IM, SC, or into body cavities; not recommended for therapy lasting longer than 10 days

- Hypoglycemia
  - PO (adults): 3–8 mg/kg/day given in divided doses, every 8–12 hr

* Cleared by hemo/peritoneal dialysis

Compatibilities
- Syringe compatibility
  - heparin
- Y-site compatibilities
  - propranolol
  - hydralazine

Adverse Effects
- Hypotension
- Tachycardia/ dysrhythmias
- CHF
- Hypoglycemia
- Angina
- Fluid/electrolyte imbalance
- Phlebitis at the IV site

Drug Interactions
- Hyperglycemia, hyperuricemia, hypotension with
  - diuretics
- Increased metabolism, decreased effectiveness of
  - phenytoin
- Increased hyperglycemia with
  - phenytoin
  - corticosteroids
  - estrogen/ progesterone

DIGOXIN (LANOXIN)

Classification: Cardiac glycoside, antidysrhythmic

Indications
Atrial fibrillation/flutter, CHF, atrial tachycardia. Therapeutic effect: slows heart rate and increases cardiac output

Contraindications
Ventricular fibrillation, AV block, idiopathic hypertrophic subaortic stenosis, constrictive pericarditis, hypersensitivity to digoxin or any of its components

Preparation/Administration	Compatibilities	Adverse Effects	Drug Interactions

• Loading dose: 0.5–1.0 mg IV or IM over 24 hr
• Maintenance dose: 0.125–0.25 mg PO/IV daily
 	
*Monitor the therapeutic drug level, which should be in the 0.8–2.0 ng/mL range
 	
*Dosage highly individualized, adjusted to clinical condition
 	
*Digoxin should be discontinued until all signs of toxicity are gone
	• Compatible with solutions containing dextrose, saline
	
	Incompatibilities
	• With all medications in syringe or solution
		• Dysrhythmias
		  – PVCs
		  – AV dissociation
		  – PAT with block
		  – severe bradycardia
		  – complete heart block
		• Hypotension
		• Headache
		• Drowsiness
		• Apathy, confusion
		• Disorientation
		• Muscle weakness
		• Photophobia
		• Agitation
		• Anorexia
		• Nausea/vomiting
		• Diarrhea
			• Potentiated by:
			  – amiodarone
			  – aminoglycosides
			  – anticholinergics
			  – quinidine
			  – quinine
			  – spironolactone
			  – verapamil
			• Antacids reduce the absorption rate of digoxin

DILTIAZEM HCL (CARDIZEM)

Classification: Calcium channel blocker, antiarrhythmic (Class IV)

Indications
Atrial fibrillation, atrial flutter, proxysmal supraventricular tachycardia (PSVT). Therapeutic effect: coronary vasodilation, decrease in frequency and severity of angina attacks

Contraindications
Sick sinus syndrome, second- or third-degree AV block (unless there is a functioning ventricular pacemaker). Severe hypotension, cardiogenic shock, demonstrated hypersensitivity to the drug. Atrial fibrillation or atrial flutter associated with WPW, or short PR syndrome. Concurrent treatment with IV beta-blockers. Patients with ventricular tachycardia

Preparation/Administration
- Initial dose 0.25 mg/kg over 2 min (20 mg is a reasonable dose for the average patient)
- Second bolus 0.35 mg/kg over 2 min (25 mg is a reasonable dose for the average patient)
- IV infusion (see chart). Infusion duration exceeding 24 hr, and infusion rate exceeding 15 mg/hr are not recommended

Compatibilities
- D_5W
- D_5/45% NaCl
- NaCl 0.9%

Adverse Effects
- Hypotension symptomatic/asymptomatic
- First- and second-degree AV block
- Bradycardia
- CHF
- Ventricular dysrhythmia
- Atrial flutter
- Chest pain
- Sinus node dysfunction
- Syncopy

Drug Interactions
- Beta-blockers
- Any agents known to affect cardiac contractility and/or SA- or AV-node conduction
- May potentiate vascular dilation associated with anesthesia
- Incompatible when mixed directly with lasix

For temporary heart-rate control during atrial fibrillation and flutter for up to 24 hr

FAST, SAFE, CONTINUOUS*
DOSING CHART BY BODY WEIGHT—BOLUS[†] OVER 2 MIN
20 mg average patient—First dose; 25 mg average patient—Second dose

Patient weight in lb	Approx weight in kg[‡]	Bolus dose at 0.25 mg/kg[§]	Bolus dose at 0.35 mg/kg[§]
90	41	10.0	14.5
100	45	11.0	16.0
110	50	12.5	17.5
120	55	13.5	19.0
130	59	14.5	20.5
140	64	16.0	22.0
150	68	17.0	24.0
160	73	18.0	25.5
170	77	19.5	27.0
180	82	20.5	28.5
190	86	21.5	30.0
200	91	22.0	31.5

*Cardizem injectable is indicated for temporary control of rapid ventricular rate during atrial fibrillation and flutter; rarely converts to normal sinus rhythm.

[†]Initial drop in B/P and/or flushing occurs during or immediately following bolus injection.

[‡]Rounded to nearest whole kg.

[§]Rounded to nearest half mg.

DILUTION/ADMINISTRATION CHART FOR CARDIZEM INJECTABLE

	Dilution		Administration	
Diluent Volume	Quantity Injectable	Final Concentration	Dose*	Infusion Rate
100 mL	125 mg (25 mL)	1.0 mg/mL	10 mg/hr	10 mL/hr
			15 mg/hr	15 mL/hr
250 mL	250 mg (50 mL)	0.83 mg/mL	10 mg/hr	12 mL/hr
			15 mg/hr	18 mL/hr
500 mL	250 mg (50 mL)	0.45 mg/mL	10 mg/hr	22 mL/hr
			15 mg/hr	33 mL/hr

*5 mg/hr may be appropriate for some patients.

IV infusions of Cardizem are predicted to produce steady-state plasma diltiazem concentrations equivalent to the total daily oral doses shown based on the results of pharmacokinetic studies in healthy volunteers administered different oral Cardizem formulations.

Based on pharmacokinetic studies in normal subjects.

The most effective and least complicated method of administering IV drugs is with tubing that delivers 60 gtts/cc.

Dosing Chart by Body Weight (September 1993) and Dilution/Administration Chart for Cardizem Injectable (November 1992) reprinted with permission from Marion Merrell Dow, Inc. (Kansas City, MO), 1995.

DOBUTAMINE HCL (DOBUTREX)

Classification: Inotropic agent

Indications
Cardiogenic shock, chronic CHF, refractory heart failure, cardiac surgery. Therapeutic effect: increased cardiac output without significant increase in heart rate

Contraindications
Hypersensitivity to the drug, sulfites, idiopathic hypertropic subaortic stenosis. **Note:** Administer cautiously to patients with atrial fibrillation, hypertension, MI, PVCs

Preparation/Administration	Compatibilities	Adverse Effects	Drug Interactions

• Initial dose: 2.5–10 mcg/ kg/min
• May increase to 40 mcg/ kg/min
• Titrate to patient response
• Dilute 250 mg in 250 mL of a compatible solution for 1000 mcg/mL
• Monitor central hemody- namics, including cardiac output, to assess clinical response to therapy
• Reconstituted solution should be used within 24 hr
	• D_5W
	• D_5/0.45% NaCl 0.9% NaCl
	• D_5 lactated Ringer's
	• Lactated Ringer's
	• NaCl 0.45% 0.9%
	• Sodium lactate ⅙ M
	• Amrinone (INOCOR)
	• Atropine
	• Dopamine
	• Epinephrine
	• Hydralazine (Apreso- line)
	• Isuprel
	• Lidocaine
	• Meperidine
		• Increased heart rate (>10%)
		• Increased B/P
		• Ventricular ectopy
		• Angina
		• Headache
		• Nausea
		• Palpitations
			• Cyclopropane, halothane
			  – ventricular dysrhythmias
			• Beta-blockers
			  – antagonize B_1 effects of dobutamine
			• Guanethidine
			  – elevates B/P and increases dysrhythmias
			• Insulin
			  – increased insulin requirements

*Infuse through central IV line using an infusion pump

*Correct hypovolemia prior to use

- Morphine
- Nipride
- Nitroglycerin
- Norepinephrine
- Pancuronium bromide
- Phenylephrine HCl
- Procainamide
- Propranolol HCl
- Ranitidine
- Streptokinase

Incompatibilities
- Alkaline solutions
- Alteplase
- Aminophyllin
- Bretylium
- Bumetamide
- Calcium chloride/ gluconate
- Digoxin
- Diazepam
- Furosemide
- Heparin
- Hydrocortisone
- Magnesium sulfate
- Phenytoin sodium
- Potassium chloride/phosphate
- Regular insulin
- Sodium bicarbonate
- Verapamil

- MAO inhibitors and tricyclic anti-depressants
  – enhance the pressor effects of dobutamine
- Nipride
  – additive effect: elevates CO_2, lowers pulmonary wedge pressure
- Rauwolfia alkaloids
  – prevents dobuta-mine uptake

Dobutamine HCl (Dobutrex) Dosage/Flow-Rate Chart[†]

Patient Weight *(lb)*	99	110	121	132	143	154	165	176	187	198	209	220
(kg)	45	50	55	60	65	70	75	80	85	90	95	100
Dosage (mcg/kg/min)												
1	3	3	3	4	4	4	5	5	5	5	6	6
2.5	7	8	8	9	10	11	11	12	13	14	14	15
5	14	15	17	18	20	21	23	24	26	27	29	30
7.5	20	23	25	27	29	32	34	36	38	41	43	45
10	27	30	33	36	39	42	45	48	51	54	57	60
12.5	34	38	41	45	49	53	56	60	64	68	71	75
15	41	45	50	54	59	63	68	72	77	81	86	90
20	54	60	66	72	78	84	90	96	102	108	114	120
30	81	90	99	108	117	126	135	144	153	162	171	180
40	108	120	132	144	156	168	180	192	204	216	228	240

[†]250 mg/250 mL (1000 mcg/mL). To infuse in microdrops/min or milliliters/hr.

The most effective and least complicated method of administering IV drugs is with tubing that delivers 60 gtts/cc.

DOPAMINE HCL (INTROPIN, DOPASTAT)

Classification: Sympathomimetic agonist

Indications
Treatment of shock, increases cardiac output, blood pressure, and urine flow. Therapeutic effect: increased cardiac output/blood pressure and improved renal blood flow

Contraindications
Uncorrected hypovolemic states, persistent tachyarrhythmia, ventricular fibrillation, or known hypersensitivity to sulfites

Preparation/Administration
- Low dose: 2.5–5.0 mcg/ kg/min
  - enhances myocardial contractility, cardiac output, renal perfusion
- Moderate dose: 5.0– 10.0 mcg/kg/min
  - increases cardiac output, pulmonary and peripheral vascular resistance
- High dose: 10.0– 50.0 mcg/kg/min
  - potent vasoconstriction with diminished renal perfusion

Do not use for IV push. Avoid extravasation.

Compatibilities
- D_5W
- D_5/0.45% NaCl 0.9% NaCl
- D_5 lactated Ringer's
- Lactated Ringer's
- NaCl 0.9%
- Aminophyllin
- Amrinone (INOCOR)
- Bretylium
- Calcium chloride
- Dobutamine
- Heparin
- Solu-Cortef/ Solu-Medrol
- Lidocaine
- Nitroglycerin
- Potassium chloride
- Verapamil

Adverse Effects
- Hypotension
- Hypertension
- Dysrhythmias
- Angina
- Tissue necrosis from extravasation
- Peripheral ischemia
- Palpitations
- Nausea/vomiting
- Headache
- Azotemia

Hypovolemia should be corrected prior to institution of dopamine therapy

Drug Interactions
- Prolong and intensify effects of dopamine
  - MAO inhibitors
- Cardiac effects of dopamine antagonized by
  - beta-blockers
- Vasopressor effects of high-dose dopamine antagonized by
  - alpha adrenergic blocking agents
- Ventricular arrhythmias and hypertension with
  - halothane or cyclopropane anesthesia (reversible with propranolol)

Drug Interactions
• May produce hypotension and bradycardia in the presence of dopamine
  – phenytoin

Dosage/Flow-Rate Chart[†]

Patient Weight (lb)	99	110	121	132	143	154	165	176	187	198	209	220
(kg)	45	50	55	60	65	70	75	80	85	90	95	100
Dosage (mcg/kg/min)												
1	2	2	2	2	2	3	3	3	3	4	4	4
2.5	4	5	5	6	6	7	7	8	8	8	9	9
5	8	9	10	11	12	13	14	15	16	17	18	19
7.5	13	14	15	17	18	20	21	23	24	25	27	28
10	17	19	21	23	24	26	28	30	32	34	36	38
15	25	28	31	34	37	39	42	45	48	51	53	56
20	34	38	41	45	49	52	56	60	64	68	71	75
25	42	47	52	56	61	66	70	75	80	84	89	94
30	51	56	62	67	73	78	84	90	96	101	107	113
35	59	66	72	79	85	92	98	105	112	118	125	131
40	68	75	83	90	98	105	113	120	128	135	143	150
45	76	84	93	101	110	118	127	135	143	152	160	169
50	84	94	103	113	122	131	141	150	159	169	178	188

[†]400 mg/250 mL (1600 mcg/mL). To infuse in microdrops/min or milliliters/hr.

The most effective and least complicated method of administering IV drugs is with a tubing that delivers 60 gtts/cc.

EPINEPHRINE HCL (ADRENALIN)

Classification: Bronchodilator, cardiac stimulant, endogenous catecholamine, alpha/beta active

Indications
Bronchodilator in symptomatic treatment of asthma and other reversible airway disease, chronic bronchitis, emphysema, treatment of anaphylaxis, cardiac arrest, treatment of open-angle glaucoma, adjunct to localize anesthesia. Therapeutic effect: bronchodilation, cardiac stimulation, vasoconstriction, localization of anesthetics

Contraindications
Hypersensitivity to sympathomimetics, bisulfites. **Note:** Use cautiously in cardiovascular disease, dysrhythmias, hypertension, hyperthyroidism, elderly patients, diabetes mellitus, pregnancy, and lactation

Preparation/Administration	Compatibilities	Adverse Effects	Drug Interactions

• Bronchodilator
  – SC/IM (adults) 1:1000 solution: 0.2–0.5 mg every 20 min (maximum dose 1 mg)
  – IV: 0.1–0.25 mg (single-dose maximum: 1 mg)
• Cardiac arrest
  – IV/intracardiac, 1:10,000 solution: 0.1–1.0 mg every 5 min as needed
  – intratracheal: 1 mg
	• D_5W
	• D_5/0.2% NaCl
	  0.45% NaCl
	  0.9% NaCl
	• D_5 Ringer's
	• D_5 lactated Ringer's
	• Ringer's
	• Lactated Ringer's
	• NaCl 0.9%
	• Amikacin
	• Amrinone
	• Calcium chloride/ gluconate
		• Hypertension
		• Dysrhythmias
		  – tachycardia
		  – reflex bradycardia
		• Pulmonary edema
		• Angina
		• CNS effects
		  – nervousness
		  – restlessness
		  – insomnia
		  – tremor
		  – headache
		• Hyperglycemia
			• Additive effect with
			  – other adrenergic agents
			  – decongestants
			• Hypertensive crisis with
			  – MAO inhibitors
			• Therapeutic response blocked by
			  – beta-adrenergic blockers
			• Increased risk of dysrhythmia with
			  – cardiac glycosides
			  – general anesthesia

Preparation/Administration

- Hypersensitivity reaction
  - SC/IM, 1:10,000 solution: 200–500 mcg every 15 min
  - dose may be increased to 1 mg
- Anaphylactic shock
  - IV (adults), 1:10,000 solution: 0.1–0.25 mg
  - slowly over 5–10 min
  - may follow with infusion of 1–4 mcg/min
  - SC/IM: 500 mcg every 5 min
  - may follow with IV infusion of 1–4 mcg/min

Compatibilities

- Cimetidine
- Dobutamine
- Doxapram
- Famotidine
- Furosemide
- Heparin
- Hydrocortisone sodium succinate
- Metaraminol bitartrate
- Pancuronium bromide
- Potassium chloride
- Vecuronium bromide
- Verapamil

Adverse Effects

- Nausea/vomiting
- Urinary retention/ hesitancy

Dosage/Flow-Rate Chart
Dilution/Concentration[†]

Dosage (mcg/min)	mL/hr or microdrops/min
0.5	7
1	15
2	30
3	45
4	60
5	75
6	90

[†]1 mg/250 mL (4 mcg/mL). To infuse in milliliters/hr or microdrops/min.

The most effective and least complicated method of administering IV drugs is with tubing that delivers 60 gtts/cc.

ESMOLOL HCL (BREVIBLOC)

Classification: Beta-blocking agent (cardioselective)

Indications
Supraventricular tachycardia, noncompensatory tachycardia, surgical hypertension, control of rapid ventricular response in atrial fibrillation/flutter. Therapeutic effect: control of ventricular response in supraventricular tach-yarrhythmias

Contraindications
Uncompensated CHF, pulmonary edema, cardiogenic shock, bradycardia, second- or third-degree heart block.
Note: Use cautiously in thyrotoxicosis, hypoglycemia, pregnancy, lactation

Preparation/Administration	Compatibilities	Adverse Effects	Drug Interactions
• *Must be diluted*	• D_5W	• Asystole	• Additive myocardial
• *Infuse into central line or large vein*	• D_5/0.45% NaCl 0.9% NaCl	• Hypotension	depression with
		• Chest pain	– verapamil
• Supraventricular	• D_5 Ringer's lactate	• Pulmonary edema	– phenytoin
tachycardia	• Lactated Ringer's	• Bronchospasm	– general anesthesia
– loading dose: 500 mcg/ kg/min (0.5 mg/kg/min); infuse for 1 min	• NaCl 0.45% 0.9%	• PVCs	• Additive bradycardia with
	• Aminophyllin	• Bradycardia	– cardiac glycosides
– maintenance dose:	• Atracurium besylate	• Phlebitis	• Additive hypotension
50 mcg/kg/min for	• Bretylium	• Pheripherial ischemia	with
4 min; *maximum*	• Calcium chloride		– alcohol
infusion rate of 300	• Cimetidine		– nitrates
mcg/kg/min	• Dopamine		
	• Heparin		
	• Hydrocortisone		
	• Magnesium sulfate		

- after 5 min, if necessary, give a second loading dose of 500 mcg/kg/min, over 1 min (0.5 mg/kg/min) followed by 100 mcg/kg/min
- Intraoperative
  - bolus dose: 1 mg/kg over 30 sec
  - followed by 150 mcg/kg/min continuous infusion if necessary
  - adjust rate, as indicated, up to 300 mcg/kg/min
- Postoperative
  - same dosing schedule as supraventricular tachycardia

Brevibloc infusions should not be abruptly discontinued; eliminate loading doses and decrease dosage by 25 mcg/kg/min

- Morphine
- Pancuronium bromide
- Potassium chloride/phosphate
- Ranitidine
- Sodium acetate
- Streptomycin
- Vecuronium bromide

Incompatibilities
- Diazepam
- Lasix
- Procainamide
- Sodium bicarbonate
- Thiopental sodium

- Excessive alpha adrenergic stimulation (hypertension/bradycardia) with
  - amphetamines
  - cocaine
  - ephedrine
  - epinephrine
  - norepinephrine
  - phenylephrine
  - pseudoephedrine
- Negates beneficial beta$_1$ effect of
  - dopamine
  - dobutamine
- Effectiveness decreased with
  - thyroid preparations
- Prolonged hypoglycemia with
  - insulin
- Potential effect of
  - succinylcholine
- Activity of Esmolol increased with morphine

Brevibloc® (Esmolol HCl) Injection
Loading Dose and Continuous Infusion Rates

Patient Weight kg (lb)	45(99)	50(110)	55(121)	60(132)	65(143)	70(154)	75(165)	80(176)	85(187)	90(198)	95(209)	100(220)
Loading Dose: 0.5 mg/kg over 1 min						Total mLs/30 sec						
	2.25	2.5	2.75	3	3.25	3.5	3.75	4	4.25	4.5	4.75	5
Followed by Infusion (Titrate to desired effect) (Range 50–300 mcg/kg/min)					Infusion Rates—Volumetric Mode (mL/h)							
50 mcg/kg/min	13.5	15	16.5	18	19.5	21	22.5	24	25.5	27	28.5	30
100 mcg/kg/min	27	30	33	36	39	42	45	48	51	54	57	60
150 mcg/kg/min	40.5	45	49.5	54	58.5	63	67.5	72	76.5	81	85.5	90
200 mcg/kg/min	54	60	66	72	78	84	90	96	102	108	114	120
250 mcg/kg/min	67.5	75	82.5	90	97.5	105	112.5	120	127.5	135	142.5	150
300 mcg/kg/min	81	90	99	108	117	126	135	144	153	162	171	180

Preparation

Add one 2.5-g ampul to 250-mL diluent (*no sodium bicarbonate*) or two 2.5-g ampuls to 500-mL diluent (*no sodium bicarbonate*); for concentration of 10 mg/mL, please see full prescribing information

The most effective and least complicated method of administering IV drugs is with tubing that delivers 60 gtts/cc.

Loading Dose and Continuous Infusion Rates, with drug preparation (1995 chart), reprinted with permission from Ohmeda Inc., Pharmaceutical Products Division (Liberty Corner, NJ), 1995.

FLECAINIDE ACETATE (TAMBOCOR)

Classification: Antiarrhythmic (Class Ic)

Indications
Supraventricular tachycardia, life-threatening ventricular dysrhythmias (including ventricular tachycardia), paroxysmal atrial fibrillation/flutter. Therapeutic effect: suppression of dysrhythmias

Contraindications
Hypersensitivity, cardiogenic shock. **Note:** Use cautiously in preexisting sinus-node dysfunction, second- or third-degree heart block (without a pacemaker); dosage reduction may be required with CHF and renal impairment. Use *cautiously* in patients with permanent or temporary pacemaker; may increase endocardial pacing thresholds. *Use extreme caution* in patients with sick sinus syndrome; may precipitate sinus bradycardia, sinus pause, or sinus arrest

Preparation/Administration	Compatibilities	Adverse Effects	Drug Interactions

• PO (adults): 50–100 mg every 12 hr initially
  – increased by 50 mg BID until response is obtained
  – maximum total dose: 400 mg
* Because of long half-life (12–72 hr), dosage adjustments should be at least 4 days apart
Monitor therapeutic blood level, range 0.2–1.0 mcg/mL
	(See Drug Interactions)	• Dysrhythmias
		• CHF
		• Bronchospasm/ dyspnea
		• Chest pain
		• Palpitations
		• EKG changes
		• Edema
		• Nausea/vomiting
		• Anorexia
		• Urinary retention
			• Additive cardiac effects with
			  – other anti- arrhythmics
			  – calcium channel blockers
			• Additive myocardial depressant effect with
			  – verapamil
			  – disopyramide
			• Increases serum digoxin levels by 15–25%

Antidysrhythmic therapy
(except lidocaine) should
be discontinued 2–4
half-lives prior to
initiating flecainide
therapy. Increases in
flecainide dosage should
be no more frequently
than every 4 days

Drug Interactions
- Increased levels of beta-adrenergic blocker and flecainide with
  - concurrent beta-adrenergic blocker therapy
- Increases flecainide blood levels, promotes reabsorption and may cause toxicity
  - alkalinizing agents
- Increased renal elimination, decreased effectiveness of flecainide (if urine pH <5)
  - acidifying agents
- Increases flecainide levels, toxicity with
  - amiodarone
    * reduced flecainide dosage recommended
- Results in increased blood levels with
  - foods that increase urine pH to >7 (i.e., strict vegetarian diet)
- Increased renal elimination, decreased effectiveness of flecainide with
  - foods or beverages that decrease urine pH to <5 (i.e., acidic juices)

FUROSEMIDE INJECTION (LASIX)

Classification: Potent diuretic (Loop diuretic)

Indications
Edema secondary to CHF, pulmonary edema, hypertensive crisis, management of hypercalcemia of malignancy. Therapeutic effect: mobilization and diuresis of excess fluid, lowers B/P

Contraindications
Hypersensitivity, cross-sensitivity with thiazides and sulfonamides, pregnancy, and lactation. **Note:** Use cautiously in electrolyte depletion, diabetes, anuria, azotemia, severe liver disease

Preparation/Administration	Compatibilities	Adverse Effects	Drug Interactions

• IM/IV (adults): 20–80 mg daily
    – up to 600 mg may be necessary
 • Continuous infusion: do not exceed 4 mg/min
	• D_5W
	 • D_5/0.9% NaCl
	 • D_5 lactated Ringer's
	 • Lactated Ringer's
	 • NaCl 0.9%
	 • Amikacin
	 • Cimetidine
	 • Cisplatin
	 • Cyclophosphamide
	 • Dexamethasone sodium phosphate
	 • Famotidine
	 • Fluorouracil
	 • Heparin
	 • Lidocaine
		• Electrolyte imbalance
		    – hyponatremia
		    – hypokalemia
		    – hypochloremia
		    – hypomagnesemia
		 • Hypovolemia/ dehydration
		 • Metabolic alkalosis
		 • CNS effects
		    – dizziness
		    – headache
		    – encephalopathy
		 • Hyperuricemia
			• Additive hypotension with
			    – antihypertensive agents
			    – nitrates
			 • Additive hypokalemia with
			    – other diuretics
			    – amphotericin
			    – mezlocillin
			    – piperacillin
			    – glucocorticoids
			     * hypokalemia may increase cardiac glycoside toxicity

- Methotrexate sodium
- Ranitidine
- Verapamil

Incompatibilities
- Diazepam
- Epinephrine
- Esmolol
- Fluconazole
- Hydralazine
- Isuprel
- Metoclopramide
- Norepinephrine
- Promethazine

- Decreased excretion of
  – lithium
- Possible ototoxicity with
  – aminoglycosides
- Increases effectiveness of
  – oral anticoagulants

ISOPROTERENOL HCL (ISUPREL)

Classification: Bronchodilator, beta-adrenergic agonist, antiarrhythmic, inotropic agent

Indications
Management of ventricular dysrhythmias secondary to AV nodal block, treatment of shock associated with vaso-constriction and decreased cardiac output, bronchodilator in reversible airway obstruction due to asthma or COPD. Therapeutic effect: increased cardiac output, increased heart rate and bronchodilator. **Note:** Stimulates β-1 (myocardial) and β-2 (pulmonary) receptors

Contraindications
Hypersensitivity to adrenergic amines, fluorocarbons, bisulfites. **Note:** Use cautiously with cardiac disease, hypertension, diabetes, glaucoma, hyperthyroidism, elderly patients, and pregnancy (near-term)

Preparation/Administration	Compatibilities	Adverse Effects	Drug Interactions

(Refer to following Dosage and Administration charts)	• D_5W
	• D_5/0.9% NaCl
	• D_5 lactated Ringer's
	• Lactated Ringer's
	• NaCl 0.9%
	• Amrinone
	• Bretylium
	• Calcium chloride/gluceptate
	• Cimetidine
	• Dobutamine
	• Famotidine
	• Heparin
	• Hydrocortisone sodium succinate
		• Angina/dysrhythmias
		• Hypotension/hypertension
		• Paradoxical bronchospasm
		• Pulmonary edema
		• CNS effects
		  – nervousness
		  – restlessness
		  – tremor
		  – insomnia
		  – headache
		• Nausea/vomiting
		• Hyperglycemia
			• Additive adrenergic effect with
			  – sympathomimetic (adrenergic) agents
			• Hypertensive crisis with
			  – MAO inhibitors
			• Therapeutic effect blocked by
			  – beta-adrenergic blockers
			• Increased arrhythmias with
			  – cyclopropane or halothane anesthesia

- Magnesium sulfate
- Pancuronium bromide
- Potassium chloride
- Ranitidine
- Succinylcholine chloride
- Vecuronium bromide
- Verapamil

Incompatibilities
- Aminophyllin
- Barbiturates
- Furosemide
- Lidocaine
- Sodium bicarbonate

- Reduced effect of antihypertensive agents
- Increased risk of dysrhythmias with
  – cardiac glycosides
- Excessive CNS stimulation with
  – CNS stimulants

Dosage and Administration

ISUPREL injection 1:5000 generally should be started at the lowest recommended dose and the rate of administration gradually increased if necessary while carefully monitoring the patient. The usual route of administration is by IV infusion or bolus IV injection. In dire emergencies, the drug may be administered by intracardiac injection. If time is not of the utmost importance, initial therapy by intramuscular or subcutaneous injection is preferred.

Recommended dosage for adults with heart block, Adams–Stokes attacks, and cardiac arrest

Route of Administration	Preparation of Dilution	Initial Dose	Subsequent Dose Range*
Bolus IV injection	Dilute 1 mL (0.2 mg) to 10 mL with sodium chloride injection, USP, or 5% dextrose injection, USP	0.02 mg to 0.06 mg (1 mL to 3 mL of diluted solution)	0.01–0.2 mg (0.5–10 mL of diluted solution)
IV infusion	Dilute 10 mL (2 mg) in 500 mL of 5% dextrose injection, USP	5 μg/min (1.25 mL of diluted solution/min)	
Intramuscular	Use solution 1:5000 undiluted	0.2 mg (1 mL)	0.02–1 mg (0.1–5 mL)
Subcutaneous	Use solution 1:5000 undiluted	0.2 mg (1 mL)	0.15–0.2 mg (0.75–1 mL)
Intracardiac	Use solution 1:5000 undiluted	0.02 mg (0.1 mL)	

*Subsequent dosage and method of administration depend on the ventricular rate and the rapidity with which the cardiac pacemaker can take over when the drug is gradually withdrawn.

Refer to full package insert for full prescribing information.

There are no well-controlled studies in children to establish appropriate dosing; however, the American Heart Association recommends an initial infusion rate of 0.1 μg/kg/min, with the usual range being 0.1–1.0 μg/kg/min.

Recommended dosage for adults with shock and hypoperfusion states

Route of Administration	Preparation of Dilution†	Infusion Rate††
IV infusion	Dilute 5 mL (1 mg) in 500 mL of 5% dextrose injection, USP	0.5–5 μg/min (0.25–2.5 mL of diluted solution

†Concentrations up to 10 times greater have been used when limitation of volume is essential.

††Rates over 30 μg/min have been used in advanced stages of shock. The rate of infusion should be adjusted on the basis of heart rate, central venous pressure, systemic blood pressure, and urine flow. If the heart rate exceeds 110 beats/min, it may be advisable to decrease or temporarily discontinue the infusion.

Refer to full package insert for full prescribing information.

Recommended dosage for adults with bronchospasm occurring during anesthesia

Route of Administration	Preparation of Dilution	Initial Dose	Subsequent Dose
Bolus IV injection	Dilute 1 mL (0.2 mg) to 10 mL with sodium chloride injection, USP, or 5% dextrose injection, USP	0.01–0.02 mg (0.5–1 mL of diluted solution)	The initial dose may be repeated when necessary

The most effective and least complicated method of administering IV drugs is with tubing that delivers 60 gtts/cc.

Refer to full package insert for full prescribing information.

Dosage and Administration charts for Isuprel injection reprinted with permission of Sanofi Winthrop Pharmaceuticals, June 1993 product information (90 Park Ave., New York, NY 10016).

Dosage/Flow-Rate Chart
Dilution/Concentration[†]

Dosage (mcg/min)	mL/hr or microdrops/min
1	15
2	30
3	45
4	60
5	75
6	90
8	120
12	180

[†]1 mg/250 mL (4 mcg/mL). To infuse in milliliters/hr or microdrops/min.

The most effective and least complicated method of administering IV drugs is with tubing that delivers 60 gtts/cc.

ISOSORBIDE DINITRATE (ISORDIL, ISOGARD)

Classification: Vasodilator, nitrate, antianginal

Indications
Acute management of angina, long-term management of angina, chronic congestive heart failure. Therapeutic effect: increased cardiac output, relief of angina

Contraindications
Severe anemia, sensitivity to nitrates. **Note:** Use cautiously in head trauma, cerebral hemorrhage, increased intracranial pressure

Preparation/Administration	Compatibilities	Adverse Effects	Drug Interactions
• PO: 5–30 mg QID – sustained release: 40 mg every 6–12 hr • SL: 2.5–10 mg; may repeat every 2–3 hr • Chewtab: 5–10 mg prn or every 2–3 hr as prophylaxis	(See Drug Interactions)	• Hypotension • Tachycardia • Headache/dizziness • Nausea/vomiting/ abdominal pain • Tolerance to this drug and cross-tolerance to other nitrates and nitrites may occur	• Additive hypotension with – antihypertensives – acute alcohol ingestion – beta-blockers – calcium channel blockers – phenothiazines • Decreased effect of Isordil with – sympathomimetics • May antagonize the anticoagulant effect of – heparin

LABETOLOL (TRANDATE, NORMODYNE)

Classification: Beta-blocker, alpha blocker, antihypertensive

Indications
Hypertension, production of controlled hypotension during surgery. Therapeutic effect: decreased heart rate and B/P

Contraindications
Asthma, bradycardia, cardiogenic shock, heart block, CHF, pulmonary edema

Preparation/Administration	Compatibilities	Adverse Effects	Drug Interactions

• PO: 100 mg BID (may be given with a diuretic)
  – may increase to 200 mg BID after 2–3 days
  – maximum dose: 400 mg BID
• IV bolus: 20 mg or 1–2 mg/kg *(whichever is the lowest dose)* over a 2-min period
  – additional dose of 40–80 mg can be given at 10-min intervals, to a total of 300 mg
	• D₅W
	• D₅/0.45% NaCl
	    0.9% NaCl
	• D₅ Ringer's
	• D₅ lactated Ringer's
	• Aminophyllin
	• Calcium gluconate
	• Cimetidine
	• Demerol
	• Dopamine
	• Heparin
	• Lidocaine
	• Magnesium sulfate
	• Morphine
	• Potassium chloride
	• Ranitidine
		• Orthostatic hypotension
		• Bradycardia
		• Bronchospasm
		• Edema
		• Paresthesia
		• Drowsiness
		• Fatigue
		• Nausea
		• Nasal congestion
			• Reflex hypertension with
			  – other antihypertensive agents
			• Potentiated by
			  – cimetidine
			• Further drop in B/P with
			  – halothane
			  – other antihypertensive agents
			  – estrogens
			  – nitrates
			  – acute alcohol ingestion

- Continuous infusion: 200 mg (40 mL) diluted in 160 mL of a compatible solution (1 mg/1 mL)
  - to be administered at 2 mg/min

Dosage is highly individualized. Abrupt withdrawal may precipitate life-threatening dysrhythmias, hypertension, or myocardial ischemia

- Increased tremors with
  - tricyclic antidepressants
- Decreased labetolol effect with
  - glutethimide
- Hypertension lasting up to 14 days after discontinuation of labetolol with
  - MAO inhibitors

METOPROLOL TARTRATE (LOPRESSOR)

Classification: Beta-blocker, antianginal, antihypertensive

Indications

Hypertension, angina, prevention of MI. Unlabeled uses: prophylaxis and treatment of dysrhythmias, treatment of mitral valve prolapse, hypertrophic cardiomyopathy, tremors, prevention of vascular headaches, symptomatic treatment of pheochromocytoma, and management of aggressive behavior. Therapeutic effect: decreased heart rate and decreased B/P

Contraindications

Cardiogenic shock, uncompensated CHF, bradycardia, heart block, pulmonary edema. **Note:** Use cautiously in hyperthyroidism, diabetes mellitus, pregnancy, and lactation

Preparation/Administration	Compatibilities	Adverse Effects	Drug Interactions

• PO (adults): 100–450 mg daily (single-dose or BID)
• IV (adults) MI prophylaxis: 5 mg every 2 min times 3 doses
  – 15 min after IV dose, a PO dose of 50 mg should be administered and repeated every 6 hr for 48 hr
  – maintenance dose of 100 mg PO, BID, thereafter
	• Dextrose solutions
	• Saline solutions
		• Bradycardia
		• CHF/pulmonary edema
		• Bronchoconstriction
		• Peripheral vasoconstriction
		• Altered glucose metabolism
		• Dizziness
		• Mental changes
		  – depression
		  – memory loss
			• Additive myocardial depression with
			  – general anesthesia
			  – phenytoin
			  – verapamil
			• Additive bradycardia with
			  – cardiac glycosides
			• Additive hypotension with
			  – nitrates
			  – other antihypertensives
			  – alcohol

- PO (adults) angina: 100 mg daily in 2 divided doses
  - usual maintenance dose is 100–400 mg daily
- PO (adults) hypotensive effect: initial 100 mg, daily in single or divided doses
  - increase at weekly intervals until optimum effect is achieved
  - maintenance dose: 100–450 mg daily

To discontinue long-term therapy, dosage of drug should be gradually reduced over 1–2 wks

Abrupt withdrawal may result in life-threatening dysrhythmias, hypertension, or myocardial ischemia

- Excessive alpha-adrenergic stimulation, hypertension, bradycardia with
  - amphetamines
  - epinephrine
  - norepinephrine
  - ephedrine
  - pseudoephedrine
  - phenylephrine
  - cocaine
- May reduce beneficial beta effects of
  - dobutamine
  - dopamine
- Decreased effectiveness with
  - thyroid preparations
- Prolonged hypoglycemia with
  - insulin

MILRINONE LACTATE (PRIMACOR® IV)

Classification: Inotropic, vasodilator

Indications
Congestive heart failure. Therapeutic effect: increased cardiac contractility and vasodilation

Contraindications
Hypersensitivity to the drug, severe obstructive aortic, pulmonic valvular disease

Preparation/Administration	**Compatibilities**	**Adverse Effects**	**Drug Interaction**

• Loading dose: 50 mcg/kg over 10 min
   – may be administered undiluted
   – diluting to a rounded total volume of 10 or 20 mL may simplify visualization of injection rate
 • Maintenance dose adjusted to hemodynamic and clinical response
   – administered as a continuous IV infusion
   – minimal dose: 0.375 mcg/kg/min (total daily/24 hr dose 0.59 mg/kg)
	• D$_5$W
	 • NaCl 0.45% 0.9%
	
	 Incompatibility
	 • Do not inject furosemide into IV lines containing PRIMACOR®
		• Ventricular dysrhythmias
		   – ectopy
		   – nonsustained/ sustained ventricular tachycardia
		   – ventricular fibrillation
		   – supraventricular dysrhythmias
		 • Angina
		 • Hypotension
		 • Hypokalemia
			• No untoward clinical manifestation in *limited* experience with
			   – digitalis glycosides
			   – lidocaine
			   – quinidine
			   – hydralazine
			   – prazosin
			   – isosorbide dinitrate

– standard dose: 0.50
mcg/kg/min (total
daily/24 hr dose 0.77
mg/kg)
– maximum dose: 0.75
mcg/kg/min (total
daily/24 dose 1.13
mg/kg)

The chart below shows the loading dose in milliliters (mL) of PRIMACOR® (1 mg/mL) by patient body weight

PRIMACOR® IV Dosing Charts
Loading Dose (mL) Using 1 mg/mL Concentration

					Patient Body Weight (kg)					
kg	30	40	50	60	70	80	90	100	110	120
mL	1.5	2.0	2.5	3.0	3.5	4.0	4.5	5.0	5.5	6.0

The loading dose may be given undiluted, but diluting to a rounded total volume of 10–20 mL may simplify the visualization of the injection rate.

Refer to full package insert for full prescribing information.

The chart below shows the volume of diluent in milliliters (mL) that must be used to achieve concentrations recommended for infusion—100 μg/mL, 150 μg/mL, or 200 μg/mL—and the resultant total volumes

Desired Infusion Concentration (μg/mL)	PRIMACOR® 1 mg/mL (mL)	Diluent (mL)	Total Volume (mL)
100	10	90	100
100	20	180	200
150	10	56.7	66.7
150	20	113	133
200	10	40	50
200	20	80	100

Refer to full package insert for full prescribing information.

The maintenance dose in mL/hr by patient body weight may be determined by reference to one of the three charts on the following two pages.

PRIMACOR® Infusion Rate (mL/hr) Using 100 µg/mL Concentration

Maintenance Dose (µg/kg/min)	Patient Body Weight (kg)									
	30	40	50	60	70	80	90	100	110	120
0.375	6.8	9.0	11.3	13.5	15.8	18.0	20.3	22.5	24.8	27.0
0.400	7.2	9.6	12.0	14.4	16.8	19.2	21.6	24.0	26.4	28.8
0.500	9.0	12.0	15.0	18.0	21.0	24.0	27.0	30.0	33.0	36.0
0.600	10.8	14.4	18.0	21.6	25.2	28.8	32.4	36.0	39.6	43.2
0.700	12.6	16.8	21.0	25.2	29.4	33.6	37.8	42.0	46.2	50.4
0.750	13.5	18.0	22.5	27.0	31.5	36.0	40.5	45.0	49.5	54.0

Refer to full package insert for full prescribing information.

PRIMACOR® Infusion Rate (mL/hr) Using 150 µg/mL Concentration

Maintenance Dose (µg/kg/min)	Patient Body Weight (kg)									
	30	40	50	60	70	80	90	100	110	120
0.375	4.5	6.0	7.5	9.0	10.5	12.0	13.5	15.0	16.5	18.0
0.400	4.8	6.4	8.0	9.6	11.2	12.8	14.4	16.0	17.6	19.2
0.500	6.0	8.0	10.0	12.0	14.0	16.0	18.0	20.0	22.0	24.0
0.600	7.2	9.6	12.0	14.4	16.8	19.2	21.6	24.0	26.4	28.8
0.700	8.4	11.2	14.0	16.8	19.6	22.4	25.2	28.0	30.8	33.6
0.750	9.0	12.0	15.0	18.0	21.0	24.0	27.0	30.0	33.0	36.0

Refer to full package insert for full prescribing information.

PRIMACOR® Infusion Rate (mL/hr) Using 200 µg/mL Concentration

Maintenance Dose	Patient Body Weight (kg)									
(µg/kg/min)	30	40	50	60	70	80	90	100	110	120
0.375	3.4	4.5	5.6	6.8	7.9	9.0	10.1	11.3	12.4	13.5
0.400	3.6	4.8	6.0	7.2	8.4	9.6	10.8	12.0	13.2	14.4
0.500	4.5	6.0	7.5	9.0	10.5	12.0	13.5	15.0	16.5	18.0
0.600	5.4	7.2	9.0	10.8	12.6	14.4	16.2	18.0	19.8	21.6
0.700	6.3	8.4	10.5	12.6	14.7	16.8	18.9	21.0	23.1	25.2
0.750	6.8	9.0	11.3	13.5	15.8	18.0	20.3	22.5	24.8	27.0

Note: PRIMACOR® supplied in 100-mL flexible containers (200 mg/mL in 5% dextrose injection) need not be diluted prior to use.

Refer to full package insert for full prescribing information.

Dosage Adjustment in Renally Impaired Patients

Creatinine Clearance (mL/min/1.73 m²)	Infusion Rate (μg/kg/min)
5	0.20
10	0.23
20	0.28
30	0.33
40	0.38
50	0.43

The most effective and least complicated method of administering IV drugs is with tubing that delivers 60 gtts/cc.

Refer to full package insert for full prescribing information.

PRIMACOR® IV Dosing Charts (Loading Dose chart, Volume of Diluent and Resultant Total Volumes chart with three Infusion Rate concentration example charts, and Dosage Adjustment in Renally Impaired Patients chart) reprinted with permission from Sanofi Winthrop Pharmaceuticals (New York), November 1994.

NADOLOL (CORGARD)

Classification: Beta-adrenergic blocker (nonselective), antihypertensive, antianginal

Indications

Treatment of angina, hypertension, prevention of myocardial infarction. Unlabeled uses: treatment of tachydysrhythmias, anxiety, aggressive behavior, migraine prophylaxis. Therapeutic effect: decreased heart rate, decreased B/P

Contraindications

Pulmonary edema, uncompensated CHF, cardiogenic shock, bradycardia, heart block, COPD, asthma, bronchospastic disease. **Note:** Use cautiously in renal impairment, thyrotoxicosis, pregnancy, and lactation

Preparation/Administration	Compatibilities	Adverse Effects	Drug Interactions

• PO (adults): 40–80 mg once daily
  – doses up to 240 mg a day have been used
 	
Abrupt withdrawal may result in life-threatening dysrhythmias, hypertension, or myocardial ischemia
 	
* Moderately dialyzable (20%–50%)
	(See Drug Interactions)	• Bradycardia
		• Bronchospasm/ wheezing
		• CHF/pulmonary edema
		• Fatigue/weakness/ drowsiness
			• Additive myocardial depression with
			  – verapamil
			  – IV phenytoin
			  – general anesthesia
			• Additive bradycardia with
			  – cardiac glycosides
			• Additive hypotension with
			  – other antihypertensive agents
			  – nitrates
			  – acute alcohol ingestion

- Decreased effective-
  ness with
  – NSAIDS
  – thyroid replacement
- Excessive alpha-
  adrenergic stimula-
  tion with
  – amphetamines
  – ephedrine
  – epinephrine
  – norepinephrine
  – phenylephrine
  – pseudoephedrine
- May produce pro-
  longed hypoglycemia
  with
  – insulin
- May produce
  hypertension with
  – MAO inhibitors
  (within 14 days of
  therapy)

NIFEDIPINE (PROCARDIA)

Classification: Calcium channel blocker

Indications

Angina (coronary artery spasm), exertional angina, hypertension. Unlabeled uses: Sublingual—acute treatment of hypertension; PO—migraine headache, Raynaud's syndrome, CHF. Therapeutic effect: coronary vasodilation, decrease in frequency/severity of attacks of angina, lowers B/P

Contraindications

Sick sinus syndrome, second- or third-degree heart block, hypotension (<90 mm Hg systolic). **Note:** Use cautiously in severe hepatic disease, CHF, edema, aortic stenosis, pregnancy, or lactation

Preparation/Administration	Compatibilities	Adverse Effects	Drug Interactions

• Initial: 10 mg, TID, maintenance 10–30 mg, 3–4 times daily
• Sustained release: 30–60 mg once daily
 	
Dosages exceeding 120-mg sustained release are not recommended. Do not chew or break sustained release capsule.
	(See Drug Interactions)	• Myocardial infarction
		• CHF
		• Hypotension
		• Dysrhythmias
		• Bradycardia
		• Tachycardia
		• Palpitations
		• Edema
		• Nausea/vomiting
		• Acute renal failure
		• Drowsiness, dizziness
		• Anxiety, confusion
			• Combined with beta-blockers
			  – increases the likelihood of CHF
			  – severe hypotension
			  – worsening of angina
			  – increased risk of bradycardia, conduction defects
			• Potentiated by cimetidine

- Antihypertensives, alcohol, or nitrates result in additive hypotension
- Cumulative effect in patients taking digitalis
- Potentiates coumarin anticoagulants
- NSAIDS may decrease anti-hypertensive effects

NITROGLYCERIN (NITRO-BID, TRIDIL)

Classification: Coronary vasodilator, nitrate

Indications
Acute angina, prophylaxis for angina, CHF, acute MI, controlled hypotension during surgical procedure. Therapeutic effect: relief or prevention of angina, increased cardiac output

Contraindications
Hypersensitivity, closed-angle glaucoma, hypotension, increased intracranial pressure, cerebral hemorrhage, constrictive pericarditis, pericardial tamponade

Preparation/Administration	Compatibilities	Adverse Effects	Drug Interactions

• Administer from glass bottle only; use non-PVC infusion sets
• Initial IV dose 5 mcg/min
  – increase by 5 mcg/min every 3–5 min
• If no response at 20 mcg/min, increase by 10–20 mcg/min until desired response obtained
• Sublingual tablets: 1 every 5 min, 3 times
	• D_5W
	• D_5/0.45% NaCl
	    0.9% NaCl
	• D_5 lactated Ringer's
	• Lactated Ringer's
	• Aminophyllin
	• Amrinone (INOCOR)
	• Dobutamine
	• Dopamine
	• Furosemide
	• Heparin
	• Lidocaine
	• Nipride
	• Pavulon
	• Ranitidine
	• Streptokinase
	• Tracrium
	• Verapamil
		• Hypotension
		• Tachycardia/ bradycardia/heart block
		• Increased angina
		• Syncopy
		• Headache
			• Potentiated by
			  – alcohol
			  – antihypertensives
			  – beta-blockers
			  – phenothiazines
			  – calcium channel blockers
			  – haldol
			• Antagonized by
			  – norepinephrine
			  – acetylcholine
			  – histamine
			
			IV NTG may antagonize the anticoagulant effect of heparin; monitor anticoagulants closely

Dosage/Flow-Rate Chart
Dilution/Concentration†

Dosage (mcg/min)	mL/hr or microdrops/min
5	–
10	3
20	6
30	9
40	12
50	15
60	18
70	21
80	24
90	27
100	30
110	33
120	36
130	39
140	42
150	45
160	48
170	51
180	54

†50 mg/250 mL (200 mcg/mL). To infuse in milliliters/hr or microdrops/min

The most effective and least complicated method of administering IV drugs is with tubing that delivers 60 gtts/cc.

NITROPRUSSIDE SODIUM (NIPRIDE, NITROPRESS)

Classification: Antihypertensive, peripheral vasodilator (arterial/venous)

Indications

Management of hypertensive crisis, control of hypertension during anesthesia, reduction of preload/afterload in cardiac pump failure, cardiogenic shock, controlled hypotension to reduce bleeding during surgery. Therapeutic effect: decreases cardiac preload and afterload, rapid lowering of B/P

Contraindications

Head trauma, cerebral hemorrhage, decreased cerebral perfusion

Preparation/Administration	Compatibilities	Adverse Effects	Drug Interactions

• IV: 0.5–10 mcg/kg/min
  – average dose of 3 mcg/kg/min
  – titrate dose to patient response
• Drug is photosensitive; container should be covered with opaque material
	• D$_5$W
	Do not mix with any drug in syringe or solution
		• May cause cyanide toxicity
		  – hypotension
		  – coma
		  – metabolic acidosis
		  – headache, dizziness
		  – dyspnea
		• Excessive hypotension
		• Substernal distress
			• Increased cardiac output, decreased PCWP with
			  – dobutamine
			• Decreased hypotensive effect with
			  – sympathomimetics
			• Additive hypotensive effect with other antihypertensive agents
			• Palpitations
			• Nausea/vomiting
			• Diaphoresis

Monitor the thiocyanate level daily if the patient is on long-term therapy. Thiocyanate is mildly neurotoxic at serum level of 1 minol/L (60 mg/L). Life-threatening when levels reach 3–4 minol/L (200 mg/L).

* Hemodialysis does not
remove cyanide; however,
it does eliminate most
thiocyanate, the
metabolite of sodium
nitroprusside

- Restlessness
- Headache
- Thyroid suppression

Dosage/Flow-Rate Chart†

Patient Weight (lb)	99	110	121	132	143	154	165	176	187	198	209	220
(kg)	45	50	55	60	65	70	75	80	85	90	95	100
Dosage (mcg/kg/min)												
0.5	–	8	8	9	10	11	11	12	13	14	14	15
1	14	15	17	18	20	21	23	24	26	27	29	30
2	27	30	33	36	39	42	45	48	51	54	57	60
3	41	45	50	54	59	63	68	72	77	81	86	90
4	54	60	66	72	78	84	90	96	102	108	114	120
5	68	75	83	90	98	105	113	120	128	135	143	150
6	81	90	99	108	117	126	135	144	153	162	171	180
7	95	105	116	126	137	147	158	168	179	189	200	210
8	108	120	132	144	156	168	180	192	204	216	228	240
9	122	135	149	162	176	189	203	216	230	243	257	270
10	135	150	165	180	195	210	225	240	255	270	285	300

†50 mg/250 mL (200 mcg/mL). To infuse in milliliters/hr or microdrops/min

The most effective and least complicated method of administering IV drugs is with tubing that delivers 60 gtts/cc.

NOREPINEPHRINE BITARTRATE (LEVOPHED)

Classification: Vasopressor, catecholamine agrenergic, alpha/beta active

Indications
Vasoconstriction, myocardial stimulation, adjunct therapy in cardiac arrest and profound hypotension, shock persisting after adequate volume replacement. Therapeutic effect: increased B/P and cardiac output

Contraindications
Thrombosis (peripheral, vascular, mesenteric), pregnancy, hypotension related to hypovolemia, hypoxia, hypercarbia, hypersensitivity to bisulfites. **Note:** Use cautiously in cardiovascular disease, hypertension, hyperthyroidism, and lactation. Use *extreme caution* when patient is on MAO inhibitors or antidepressants such as triptyline or imipramine

Preparation/Administration	Compatibilities	Adverse Effects	Drug Interactions
• For IV infusion only	• D$_5$W	• Hypertension	• Increased myocardial
• Use antecubital or femoral vein	• D$_5$/0.9% NaCl	• Cardiac dysrhythmias	irritability with
• IV: 8–12 mcg/min titrated to B/P	• Lactated Ringer's	• Metabolic acidosis	– cardiac glycosides
• Mix 2 mg in 250 mL of a compatible solution (8 mcg/mL)	*Administration in saline solution alone is not recommended	• Chest pain	– doxapram
• Discolored or precipitated solution should be discarded	• Amrinone	• Respiratory distress	– cyclopropane/halothane anesthesia
	• Calcium chloride/gluceptate/gluconate	• Peripheral ischemia, tissue hypoxia, tissue necrosis at injection site	– cocaine
Avoid extravasation	• Cimetidine	• Plasma volume depletion	• Severe hypertension when used with
	• Corticotropin	• Renal failure	– doxapram
	• Dobutamine	• Anxiety/headache	– MAO inhibitors
	• Famotidine	• Restlessness/insomnia	– guanethidine
	• Heparin	• Dizziness/weakness	– methyldopa
	• Magnesium sulfate		– tricyclic depressants
	• Potassium chloride		• Interferes with pressor

- Solu-Medrol
- Succinylcholine chloride
- Verapamil

Incompatibilities
- Aminophyllin
- Lidocaine
- Phentobarbital
- Sodium phenytoin
- Sodium bicarbonate
- Streptomycin

- – alpha-adrenergic blockers
- Enhances hypertension, blocks cardiac stimulation with
  - – beta-adrenergic blockers
- Enhanced vasoconstriction with
  - – ergotamine
  - – ergonovine
  - – methylergonovine
  - – methylsergide
  - – oxytocin

Dosage/Flow-Rate Chart
Dilution/Concentration[†]

Dosage (mcg/min)	mL/hr or microdrops/min
1	8
2	15
3	23
4	30
5	38
6	45
7	53

[†]2 mg/250 mL (8 mcg/mL). To infuse in milliliters/hr or microdrops/min

The most effective and least complicated method of administering IV drugs is with tubing that delivers 60 gtts/cc.

PHENYLEPHRINE HCL (NEO-SYNEPHRINE)

Classification: Vasopressor, sympathomimetic, adrenergic, alpha I

Indications
Shock states without blood loss, drug-induced hypotension, PSVT, hypersensitivity reaction, adjunct to spinal or general anesthesia. Therapeutic effect: increased B/P

Contraindications
Tachydysrhythmias, severe hypertension, uncorrected fluid volume deficit, hypersensitivity to phenylephrine or any of its components, pheochromocytoma, angle-closure glaucoma. **Note:** Use cautiously in cardiovascular disease, hyperthyroidism, diabetes mellitus, occlusive vascular disease, elderly patients, and during pregnancy/lactation

Preparation/Administration	Compatibilities	Adverse Effects	Drug Interactions

• IV push: 0.1% solution (1 mg/mL) 0.1–0.5 mg; usually 0.2 mg
• For PSVT:
  – rapid IV injection (20–30 sec)
• **Mix 10 mg (1 mL) in 9 mL of sterile water for injection**
• **IV push should not be administered more frequently than every 10–15 min**
	• D_5W
	• D_5/0.2% NaCl
	  0.45% NaCl
	  0.9% NaCl
	• D_5 Ringer's
	• D_5 lactated Ringer's
	• Ringer's
	• Lactated Ringer's
	• NaCl 0.45%
	  0.9%
	• Amrinone (INOCOR)
	• Dobutamine
	• Famotidine
	• Lidocaine
		• Hypertension
		• Cardiac dysrhythmias
		  – tachycardia
		  – bradycardia
		• Respiratory distress/dyspnea
		• Chest pain
		• Phlebitis/necrosis at IV site
		• Vasoconstriction
		• Dizziness/headache
		• Restlessness/weakness
		• Anxiety/nervousness
			• Severe hypotension with
			  – MAO inhibitors
			  – ergot alkaloids
			  – oxytocics
			• Myocardial irritability with
			  – general anesthetics
			• Antagonized pressor effect with
			  – alpha-adrenergic blockers (i.e., phenoxybenzmine, phentolamine)

- IV infusion: 10 mg added to 500 mL of a compatible solution
  - initially 100–180 mcg/min
  - maintenance 40–60 mcg/min
- Additional increments may be added if response is not promptly noted
- Discard discolored or precipitated solutions
- **Avoid extravasation**

- Potassium chloride
- Sodium bicarbonate
- Zidovudine

* Atropine blocks bradycardia from phenylephrine and enhances pressor effects

Dosage/Flow-Rate Chart[†]

Dilution/Concentration Infusion Rate (microdrops/min or mL/hr)	30 mg/500 mL (60 mcg/mL)	500 mg/500 mL 100 mcg/mL)
1	1.0	1.7
5	5.0	8.3
10	10.0	16.7
50	50.0	83.3
100	100.0	166.7
150	150.0	−
180	180.0	−

[†]Dosage given in mcg/min.

The most effective and least complicated method of administering IV drugs is with tubing that delivers 60 gtts/cc.

PHENYTOIN (DILANTIN)

Classification: Anticonvulsant, antiarrhythmic (Class Ib)

Indications
Prevention and treatment of tonic–clonic (grand mal) seizures, complex partial seizures, arrhythmias associated with cardiac glycoside toxicity, management of painful syndromes, including trigeminal neuralgia. Therapeutic effect: control of dysrhythmias, diminished seizure activity, decreased pain

Contraindications
Hypersensitivity to hydantoin products, sinus bradycardia, sino-atrial block, second- and third-degree AV block, Adams–Stokes syndrome

Preparation/Administration
- **IV administration not to exceed 50 mg/min**
- Status epilepticus: IV (adult) 150–250 mg (15–18 mg/kg)
  – rate not to exceed 25–50 mg/min
- Antiarrhythmic: IV (adult) 100 mg every 5 min or 50–100 mg every 10–15 min until dysrhythmia subsides
  – not to exceed 1 g
- **Not for continuous infusion**

Compatibilities
- **Phenytoin has been found to form crystals when diluted with *any* IV solution. These crystals form more rapidly in dextrose solutions and less rapidly in normal saline**
- Esmolol HCl
- Famotidine
- Fluconazole
- Foscarnet sodium
- Verapamil

Adverse Effects
- Blood dyscrasias
  – aplastic anemia
  – agranulocytosis
- Stevens–Johnson syndrome/rashes, exfoliative dermatitis
- Hypotension (IV only)
- Cardiovascular collapse
- Cardiac dysrhythmias/ bradycardia
- Pain/necrosis at IV site
- CNS effect, including coma

Drug Interactions
- Drugs that may increase serum level of phenytoin
  – chloramphenical
  – dicumarol
  – disulfiran
  – tolbutamide
  – isoniazid
  – phenylbulazone
  – cimetidine
  – acute alcohol intake
  – salicylates
  – chlormethyl- phenidate
  – phenothiazines
  – diazepam

Preparation/Administration
- **Flush line with sterile saline before and after administration**
- PO (Adult) 100 mg, 2–4 times daily

Monitor therapeutic drug level, range: 10–20 ug/mL; a relatively small margin exists between the therapeutic level and minimally toxic doses of this drug

Adverse Effects
- GI effect
  - nausea/vomiting
  - anorexia
  - constipation
  - hepatitis
- Osteomalacia

Drug Interactions
  - estrogens
  - ethosuximide
  - halothane
  - methylphenidate
  - sulfonamides
  - trazodone
- Drugs that may decrease serum level of phenytoin
  - carbamazepine
  - chronic alcohol abuse
  - reserpine
  - Moban® brand of molindone hydro-chloride
- Drugs that may either increase or decrease serum level of pheny-toin
  - phenobarbital
  - valproic acid
  - sodium valproate (activity unpre-dictable)

- Tricyclic antidepres-
  sants may precipitate
  seizures in some
  patients
- Drugs whose efficacy
  is impaired by
  phenytoin
  – corticosteroids
  – coumarin anti-
    coagulants
  – quinidine
  – vitamin D
  – digitoxin
  – rifampin
  – doxycycline
  – estrogens
  – furosemide
- May cause additive
  hypotension
  – dopamine
- Oral absorption may
  be decreased by
  antacids
- May decrease the
  absorption of folic
  acid

POTASSIUM CHLORIDE (KCL)

Classification: Electrolyte

Indications
Potassium deficiency, treatment of dysrhythmia of cardiac glycoside toxicity. Therapeutic effect: replacement of potassium in deficiency states, prevention of deficiency

Contraindications
Hyperkalemia, severe renal impairment, untreated Addison's disease, severe tissue trauma

Preparation/Administration	Compatibilities	Adverse Effects	Drug Interactions
Must be diluted before administration	• D_5W	• Cardiac arrest	• If used with potassium-spacing diuretics or ACE inhibitors, may result in hyperkalemia
• Serum potassium level *less than 2.0 mEq/liter* with EKG changes and/or muscle paralysis	• $D_{10}W$	• Cardiac dysrhythmias	
	• D_5/0.2% NaCl 0.45% NaCl 0.9% NaCl	• Dyspnea	• Captopril and enalapril may cause hyperkalemia
	• D_5 Ringer's	• Pain and phlebitis at injection site	
– may be infused, **very cautiously,** at a rate of up to 40 mEq/hr	• D_5 lactated Ringer's	• Paresthesias, weakness	
– must be administered per central line	• Ringer's	• Anxiety	
	• Lactated Ringer's	• Confusion	
Continuous cardiac monitoring is essential	• NaCl 0.45% 0.9%	• Fatigue	
– in a 24-hr period, as much as 400 mEq may be administered	**Potassium is compatible with most drugs and solutions except:**		
	– **fat emulsions**		
	– **mannitol**		
	– **diazepam**		

- Serum potassium level
  greater than 2.5 mEq/liter
  – may be administered IV
    in a concentration of up
    to 40 mEq/liter, at a rate
    not to exceed 10
    mEq/hr
  – total 24-hr dose should
    not exceed 200 mEq
- Unless contraindicated,
  and in critical conditions,
  potassium chloride may
  be administered in saline
  rather than in dextrose-
  containing fluids
  – dextrose may lower
    serum potassium levels

Potassium therapy should be guided primarily by serial ECGs, especially in individuals receiving digitalis. Tissue potassium levels are not necessarily reflected by serum potassium levels

*Continuous monitoring and infusion pump/controller required

*In cases of hyperkalemia, hemo/peritoneal dialysis may be indicated

PROCAINAMIDE HCL (PRONESTYL)

Classification: Antiarrhythmic (Class Ia)

Indications
Cardiac dysrhythmias including: premature atrial contractions, paroxysmal atrial tachycardia, premature ventricular contractions, ventricular tachycardia, atrial fibrillation. **Note:** May be ordered for malignant hyperthermia. Therapeutic effect: suppression of dysrhythmias

Contraindications
Second- or third-degree AV block, atypical ventricular tachycardia (torsades de pointes). **Note:** Use cautiously with CHF, cardiac glycoside toxicity, myocardial infarction, hepatic or renal impairment, bronchial asthma, myasthenia gravis, systemic lupus

Preparation/Administration	Compatibilities	Adverse Effects	Drug Interactions
• IV bolus: 100 mg at 25–50 mg/min, every 5 min – *do not exceed 50 mg/min* – *do not exceed 1000 mg* • Maintenance dose 2–6 mg/min – dilute 1 g in 250 mL D$_5$W (4 mg/mL) – adjust infusion rate by 1 mg/min as required for dysrhythmia control – titrated to patient response	• D$_5$W • Sterile water for injection • Physically compatible with – atropine – dobutamine – heparin – lidocaine – potassium chloride – verapamil	• Hypotension • Ventricular dysrhythmias/asystole • Tachycardia • Heart block • Agranulocytosis • Anorexia • Confusion/depression • Fatigue • Lightheadedness • Nausea/vomiting/diarrhea • Pruritis/rash	• Additive/antagonistic effect with – antiarrhythmics • Additive hypotension with – antihypertensive agents • Intensified atropine-like effect with – antihistamines – antimuscarinics – antidyskinetics (atropine, etc.) • Decreased effect of these drugs – antimyasthenics

Therapeutic drug levels should be monitored. The therapeutic range is 3–10 mcg/mL; NAPA 5–25 mcg/mL.

Monitor for prolonged QT interval.

Dosage/Flow-Rate Chart
Dilution/Concentration[†]

Dosage (mcg/min)	mL/hr or microdrops/min
1	15
2	30
3	45
4	60
5	75
6	90
7	105
8	120

[†]1000 mg/250 mL (4 mg/mL). To infuse in milliliters/hr or microdrops/min.

The most effective and least complicated method of administering IV drugs is with tubing that delivers 60 gtts/cc.

Drug Interactions

- Antagonistic cholinergic effect with
  – bethanechol
- Enhanced effect of these drugs
  – neuromuscular blocking agents
- Increased CNS effect with
  – lidocaine
- Diminished inotropic effect, potentiated hypotension with
  – bretylium
- Elevated serum pro-cainamide level with
  – cimetidine
- Increased risk of dysrhythmia
  – pimozide
- Increased leukopenia/thrombocytopenia with
  – bone marrow depressants

PROPRANOLOL HCL (INDERAL)

Classification: Antihypertensive, antianginal, nonselective beta-blocker

Indications

Hypertension, chronic stable angina, supraventricular dysrhythmias, tachycardias precipitated by thyrotoxicosis, cardiac dysrhythmias, persistent PVCs, myocardial infarction, migraine. Therapeutic effect: decreased heart rate, B/P, and AV conduction

Contraindications

Known hypersensitivity, patients with Raynaud's syndrome, malignant hypertension, bronchial asthma, sinus bradycardia, heart block greater than first degree, CHF, myocardial infarction with compromised systolic pressure, cardiogenic shock, myasthenia gravis

Preparation/Administration	Compatibilities	Adverse Effects	Drug Interactions

• Hypertension:
  – initial, PO, 10 mg QID
  – maintenance: 160–480 mg/day in 2–3 divided doses
• Angina:
  – initial, PO, 10–20 mg 3–4 times a day
  – maintenance: 160–240 mg/day
• Tachydysrhythmias:
  – PO: 30–120 mg/day, 3–4 doses daily
  – IV: 0.5–3.0 mg, no faster than 1 mg/min, may repeat in 2 min; no
	• D₅W
	• NaCl 0.9%
	
	*No incompatibilities have been reported
		• Bradycardia
		• CHF/pulmonary edema
		• Hypotension
		• Bronchospasm/ wheezing
		• Edema
		• GI disturbances
		• Hyperglycemia/ hypoglycemia
		• Neurologic disturbances
		  – drowsiness
		  – confusion
		  – mental changes
		  – memory loss
			• Additive myocardial depression with
			  – IV dilantin
			  – verapamil
			  – general anesthesia
			• Additive bradycardia with
			  – cardiac glycosides
			• Additive hypotension with
			  – antihypertensive agents
			  – nitrates
			  – acute alcohol ingestion

- Prophylaxis of myocardial infarction:
  - PO: 180–240 mg/day, 2–4 divided doses

Abrupt withdrawal may precipitate life-threatening dysrhythmias, hypertension, or ischemia

- Hypertension/bradycardia with
  - amphetamines
  - cocaine
  - epinephrine
  - norepinephrine
  - ephedrine
  - phenylephrine
  - pseudoephedrine
- Negates beta$_1$ cardiac effect of
  - dopamine
  - dobutamine
- Prolongs hypo-glycemia with
  - insulin
- Decreased antihyper-tensive effect with
  - NSAIDS
- Antagonizes beta adrenergic bronchodilators
- Increased effect of propranolol with
  - cimetidine

QUINIDINE (SULFATE: QUINORA, QUINIDEX; GLUCONATE: QUINAGLUTE, QUINALAN)

Classification: Antiarrhythmic (Class Ia)

Indications
Premature atrial contractions, premature ventricular contractions, ventricular tachycardia, paroxysmal atrial tachycardia, maintenance of regular sinus rhythm after conversion of atrial fib/flutter. Therapeutic effect: suppression of dysrhythmias

Contraindications
Cardiac glycoside toxicity, conduction defects, hypersensitivity. **Note:** Use cautiously in CHF, lactation, pregnancy, or severe liver disease (dosage reduction may be necessary)

Preparation/Administration
Quinidine sulfate (83% Quinidine)
- Premature atrial or ventricular contractions
  - PO (adult): 200–300 mg every 6–8 hr or 300–600 mg of extended-release preparation every 8–12 hr as a maintenance dose (not to exceed 4 g/day)
- Paroxysmal atrial tachycardia

Compatibilities
- D_5W
- Bretylium
- Cimetidine
- Verapamil
- Y-site compatibility
  - diazepam

Y-Site Incompatibilities
- Furosemide
- Amiodarone
- Iodide salts

Adverse Effects
- Hypotension
- Dysrhythmias
  - PVCs
  - ventricular tachycardia
  - ventricular fib/flutter
  - torsades de pointes
  - widening of QRS complex
  - prolongation of QT interval
  - complete AV block
- Arterial embolism
- Hypersensitivity
  - angioedema
  - acute asthma

Drug Interactions
- Increased serum digoxin levels (dosage reduction recommended)
- Risk of additive cardiac effects with
  - lidocaine
  - procainamide
  - phenytoin
  - propranolol
- Increased metabolism, decreased effectiveness with
  - phenytoin
  - rifampin
  - phenobarbital

- PO (adult): 400–600 mg every 2–3 hr until dysrhythmia terminates; then 200–300 mg every 6–8 hr or 300–600 mg of extended-release preparation every 8–12 hr as a maintenance dose (not to exceed 4 g/day)
- Conversion of atrial fibrillation
  - PO (adult): 200 mg every 2–3 hr for 5–8 doses. Dose may be increased daily as needed, then 200–300 mg every 6–8 hr or 300–600 mg of extended-release preparation every 8–12 hr as a maintenance dose (not to exceed 4 g/day)

- vascular collapse
- respiratory arrest
- GI effects
  - diarrhea
  - nausea
  - cramping
  - anorexia
- CNS effects
  - headache
  - dizziness
  - vertigo
- Thrombocytopenia
- Hemolytic anemia

- Decreased metabolism, increased blood level with
  - cimetidine
- Potentiates
  - oral anticoagulants
  - neuromuscular blocking agents
- Additive hypotension with
  - bretylium
  - nitrates
  - antihypertensives
  - acute alcohol ingestion
- Antagonizes
  - anticholinesterase therapy in patients with *myasthenia gravis*
- Increased risk of toxicity with
  - drugs that alkalinize urine (i.e., sodium bicarbonate)
  - high-dose antacid therapy

Preparation/Administration

Quinidine gluconate (62% Quinidine)

- PO (adult): 324–660 mg every 6–12 hr of extended release tablets
- IM (adult): 600 mg initially, up to 400 mg every 2 hr
- IV (adult) intermittent infusion: 800 mg of quinidine **gluconate** (10 mL) diluted in 40 mL D_5W for injection (maximum concentration of 16 mg/mL). Solution stable for 24 hr at room temperature
  – administer at a rate not to exceed 1 mL/min

Monitor therapeutic blood level: 3–6 mcg/mL

*Dialyzable slightly (5%–20%)

Drug Interactions

- Foods that alkalinize urine may increase serum quinidine levels and risk of toxicity (i.e., all fruit, except cranberries, prunes, plums; all vegetables and milk)

SODIUM BICARBONATE (NaHCO$_3$)

Classification: Alkalinizing agent (base)

Indications
Metabolic acidosis, alkalinizing agent in ACLS, certain intoxications (methyl alcohol, phenobarbital, salicylates), hemolytic reactions requiring alkalinization of urine to diminish nephrotoxicity of blood pigments, hyperkalemia. Therapeutic effect: alkalinization, neutralization of gastric acid

Contraindications
Metabolic/respiratory alkalosis, hypertension, hypocalcemia, hypochloremia, edema, CHF, peptic ulcer renal disease

Preparation/Administration
- In cardiac arrest
  - 1 mEq/kg initially
  - repeat at 10-min intervals with 0.5 mEq/kg
- Metabolic acidosis: 2–5 mEq/kg as a 4–8-hr infusion

Monitor serum electrolytes and ABGs.

Compatibilities
- D$_5$W
- D$_5$/0.2% NaCl
  0.45% NaCl
  0.9% NaCl
- D$_5$ Ringer's
- NaCl 0.45%
  0.9%
- Aminophyllin
- Atropine
- Bretylium
- Cimetidine
- Lasix
- Lidocaine
- Heparin
- Phenobarbital
- Phenylephrine

Adverse Effects
- Seizures/loss of consciousness
- Fluid retention
- Tissue necrosis from extravasation
- Alkalosis
- Tetany
- Gastric distention

Drug Interactions
- Potentiates
  - quinidine
  - mexiletine
  - flecainide
  - amphetamines

STREPTOKINASE (STREPTASE, KABIKINASE®)

Classification: Thrombolytic agent

The risks of streptokinase therapy may be increased and should be weighed against anticipated benefits under the following conditions:

- Recent (within 10 days)
  - major surgery
  - obstetrical delivery
  - organ biopsy
  - previous puncture of noncompressible vessels
  - serious GI bleeding
  - trauma (including CPR)
- Hypertension
  - systolic ≥180 mm Hg
  - diastolic ≥110 mm Hg
- High likelihood of left-heart thrombus (e.g., mitral stenosis with atrial fibrillation)
- Subacute bacterial endocarditis
- Hemostatic defects, including those secondary to severe hepatic or renal disease
- Cerebrovascular disease
- Pregnancy
- Age >75 years
- Diabetic hemorrhagic retinopathy
- Septic thrombophlebitis or occluded AV cannula at seriously infected site
- Any other condition in which bleeding constitutes a significant hazard or would be particularly difficult to manage because of its location

Indications

Acute evolving transmural myocardial infarction, lysis of intracoronary thrombi, improvement of ventricular function and reduction of mortality associated with AMI, reduction of infarct size, resolution of CHF associated with AMI, pulmonary embolism, deep-vein thrombosis, arterial thrombosis and embolism originating from other than left side of heart, management of occluded arteriovenous cannulae. Therapeutic effect: preservation of left ventricular function following transmural myocardial infarction, lysis of thrombi or emboli

Actions

Activates plasmogen, which subsequently dissolves fibrin deposits, **including** those required for normal hemostatis

Contraindications

Hypersensitivity to Streptase, active internal bleeding, recent (within 2 months) cerebral vascular accident, intracranial or intraspinal surgery, intracranial neoplasm, severe uncontrolled hypertension. **Precaution:** recent streptococcal infection or previous administration of Streptase may precipitate formation of an antistreptokinase antibody. Therapy may not be effective between 5 days and 6 months of such an occurrence

Pretreatment Lab

Activated partial thromboplastin time (APTT), prothrombin time (PT), thrombin time (TT), fibrinogen level, hematocrit, and platelet count. *If heparin has been administered, it should be discontinued before initiating thrombolytic therapy, and the TT or APTT should be less than twice the normal control value.*

Preparation/Administration	Compatibilities	Adverse Effects	Drug Interactions

• Avoid invasive procedures
  – if arterial/venipuncture must be performed, apply pressure to site for 30 min
  – avoid noncompressible vessels
	• D_5W
	• NaCl 0.9%
	
	Do not admix or administer Y-site injection of Streptase with any other medication
		• Bleeding
		• Reperfusion dysrhythmias
		• Anaphylactic/ anaphylactoid reactions
		• Hypotension
		• Bronchospasm
			• Increased risk of bleeding with concurrent use of
			  – other anticoagulants
			  – cefamandole
			  – cefotetan
			  – moxalactam
			  – plicamycin

Preparation/Administration

- *Reconstitution:* slowly add 5 mL of a compatible solution to the Streptase vial
  - direct the diluent at the side of vial
  - do not direct diluent into the drug powder
- Roll and tilt vial gently to reconstitute
  - avoid shaking (may cause foaming)
- *Dilution:* withdraw entire contents of vial and further dilute to a total volume as recommended in Table 8-1
  - avoid shaking and agitation of solution
  - if necessary, total volume can be increased to a maximum of 500 mL in glass or 50 mL in plastic containers (infusion pump rate shown in Table 8-1 should be adjusted accordingly, as indicated in lab studies by Hoechst–Roussel Pharmaceuticals)
- When diluting the 1,500,000 IU infusion bottle (50 mL), slowly add 5 mL of a compatible solution
  - do not direct diluent into the drug powder
  - roll and tilt vial gently to reconstitute; avoid shaking (may cause foaming)
  - add another 40 mL of diluent to the bottle; avoid shaking and agitation (Total Volume = 45 mL); refer to Table 8-1 for indicated infusion pump rate

Adverse Effects

- Fever
- Periorbital edema
- Urticaria/flushing
- Phlebitis at IV site
- Angioneurotic edema

Drug Interactions

- agents affecting platelet function including
  - aspirin
  - dipyridamole
  - nonsteroidal anti-inflammatory agents

- Reconstituted solution may have slight yellow color
  - solution can be filtered through a 0.8-μm or larger pore size filter
- Reconstitute immediately before use
  - solution should be stored at 2–8°C (36–46°F) and used within 8 hr
- Arteriovenous cannulae occlusion:
  - slowly administer 250,000 IU of Streptase, in 2 mL of a compatible solution, into each occluded limb of the cannula
  - clamp off limb of cannula for 2 hr
  - after treatment, aspirate contents of infused cannula limb(s), flush with saline then reconnect cannula
- Following termination of streptokinase therapy, continuous IV heparin (without a loading dose) has been recommended
  - heparin therapy without a loading dose can be initiated when the TT or APTT is less than twice the normal control value

Indication	Loading Dose	IV Infusion—Dosage/Duration
Pulmonary embolism	250,000 IU/30 min	100,000 IU/hr for 24 hr (72 hr if concurrent DVT is suspected)
Deep-vein thrombosis	250,000 IU/30 min	100,000 IU/hr for 72 hr
Arterial thrombosis or embolism	250,000 IU/30 min	100,000 IU/hr for 24-72 hr

Table 8-1   Suggested Dilutions and Infusion Rates

Dosage	Vial Size (IU)	Total Solution Volume	Infusion Rate

I. Acute Myocardial
   Infarction
   A. IV Infusion
	1,500,000	45 mL	Infuse 45 mL
			within 60 min

B. Intracoronary
     Infusion
     1. 20,000 IU bolus
     2. 2,000 IU/min
       for 60 min
	250,000	125 mL	1. Loading dose
			    of 10 mL
			2. Then 60 mL/hr

II. Pulmonary Embolism,
    Deep-Vein Thrombosis,
    Arterial Thrombosis, or
    Embolism
    A. Intravenous Infusion
      1. 250,000 IU loading
        dose over 30 min
      2. 100,000 IU/hr
        maintenance dose
	1,500,000	90 mL	1. Infuse 30 ml/hr
			    for 30 min
			2. Infuse 6 mL/hr

B. Same	1,500,000 infusion bottle	45 mL	1. 15 mL/hr for 30 min 2. Infuse 3 mL/hr

VECURONIUM BROMIDE (NORCURON®)

Classification: Neuromuscular blocking agent (Nondepolarizing)

Indications
Adjunct to general anesthesia, facilitate endotracheal intubation, skeletal muscle relaxation during surgery, increased pulmonary compliance during mechanical ventilation. Therapeutic effect: skeletal muscle paralysis.

Vecuronium bromide should be administered only by individuals experienced in endotracheal intubation.

Routine use of a sedative capable of inducing unawareness (e.g., diazepam) should be administered prior to and during paralysis.

Contraindications
Hypersensitivity to the drug. **Note:** Use cautiously in patients with pulmonary or cardiovascular disease, renal or liver impairment, elderly or debilitated patients, electrolyte disturbances, myasthenic syndrome

Preparation/Administration	Compatibilities	Adverse Effects	Drug Interactions

• IV bolus injection (initial dose): 0.08–0.10 mg/kg
  – reconstitute dose in 5–10 mL of bacteriostatic water for injection
  – titrate dose according to patient response
• Continuous infusion
  – reconstitute with bacteriostatic water for injection
	• D_5W
	• D_5/0.9% NaCl
	• NaCl 0.9%
	• Lactated Ringer's
	• Sterile water for injection
		• Apnea
		• Respiratory insufficiency
		• Prolonged muscle weakness
		• Allergic reaction
			• Paralysis intensified by
			  – succinylcholine
			  – general anesthesia
			  – aminoglycoside
			  – polymyxin B
			  – lidocaine
			  – quinidine
			  – procainamide
			  – beta-blockers
			  – potassium losing diuretics

Preparation/Administration
- reconstitute 10 mg of Norcuron in 10 mL of diluent (1:1)
- dilute above solution in 100 mL of compatible IV fluids
• Maintenance dose: 0.8–1.2 mcg/kg/min

No known effect on consciousness, pain perception, anxiety states, cerebration. Neuromuscular block should be induced after patient is rendered unconscious.

Drug Interactions
- magnesium
- verapamil
• Additive neuromuscular blockade with
- inhalation anesthetics such as enflurane, isoflurane, or halothane

Infusion rates of Norcuron® can be individualized for each patient using the following table:

Drug Delivery Rate (μg/kg/min)	Infusion Delivery Rate (mL/kg/min)	
	0.1 mg/mL*	0.2 mg/mL†
0.7	0.007	0.0035
0.8	0.008	0.0040
0.9	0.009	0.0045
1.0	0.010	0.0050
1.1	0.011	0.0055
1.2	0.012	0.0060
1.3	0.013	0.0065

*10 mg of Norcuron® in 100-mL solution

†20 mg of Norcuron® in 100-mL solution

The following table is a guideline for mL/min delivery for a solution of 0.1 mg/mL (10 mg in 100 mL) with an infusion pump:

NORCURON® Infusion Rate—mL/min

Amount of Drug µg/kg/min	Patient Weight (kg)						
	40	50	60	70	80	90	100
0.7	0.28	0.35	0.42	0.49	0.56	0.63	0.70
0.8	0.32	0.40	0.48	0.56	0.64	0.72	0.80
0.9	0.36	0.45	0.54	0.63	0.72	0.81	0.90
1.0	0.40	0.50	0.60	0.70	0.80	0.90	1.00
1.1	0.44	0.55	0.66	0.77	0.88	0.99	1.10
1.2	0.48	0.60	0.72	0.84	0.96	1.08	1.20
1.3	0.52	0.65	0.78	0.91	1.04	1.17	1.30

Note: If a concentration of 0.2 mg/mL is used (20 mg in 100 mL), the rate should be decreased by one-half.
*To determine the rate of delivery, per hour, **in mL,** multiply mL/min times 60.*

The most effective and least complicated method of administering IV drugs is with tubing that delivers 60 gtts/cc.

VERAPAMIL HCL (CALAN, ISOPTIN)

Classification: Calcium channel blocker, antianginal, antihypertensive, antiarrhythmic (Class IV), coronary vasodilator

Indications

Angina, management of hypertension, control of supraventricular tachydysrhythmias, atrial fibrillation, atrial flutter with rapid ventricular response. Unlabeled uses: management of hypertropic cardiomyopathy, migraine headache. Therapeutic effect: decreases severity and frequency of angina pectoris secondary to coronary dilation, decreased B/P, and suppression of supraventricular tachyarrhythmias

Contraindications

Severe hypotension, sinus bradycardia, severe congestive heart failure, advanced heart block, ventricular tachycardia, sick sinus syndrome, WPW, or known sensitivity to the drug

Preparation/Administration	Compatibilities	Adverse Effects	Drug Interactions
• IV bolus (adult): 5–10 mg over 2 min – may repeat in 30 min • PO (adult): 80 mg 3– 4 times daily or 100– 240 mg/day of extended release preparation	• D_5W • D_5 Ringer's • D_5 lactated Ringer's • Ringer's • Lactated Ringer's • NaCl 0.45% 0.9% • Aminophyllin • Amrinone lactate • Atropine • Bretylium	• Sinus arrest/asystole • Hypotension • AV block (first-, second-, or third- degree) • CHF/pulmonary edema • Edema • Bradycardia • Constipation • Nausea	• Increases serum digoxin level • Increases risk of CHF, dysrhythmias, bradycardia – beta-blockers – disapyramide • Additive hypotension – antihypertensive agents – quinidine

Compatibilities
- Calcium chloride/ gluconate
- Cimetidine
- Decadron
- Diazepam
- Digoxin
- Dopamine
- Epinephrine
- Furosemide
- Heparin
- Insulin
- Isuprel
- Lidocaine
- Magnesium sulfate
- Meperidine
- Methyldopa
- Metoclopramide
- Morphine
- Naloxone
- Nitroglycerin
- Norepinephrine
- Pancuronium
- Phenobarbital
- Phenytoin
- Potassium chloride/phosphate

Adverse Effects
- Abdominal discomfort
- Headache/dizziness
- Anxiety/depression
- Confusion

Drug Interactions
- nitrates
- alcohol
- Increases muscular relaxant effect of
  - nondepolarizing neuromuscular blockers
  - atracurium
  - doxacurium
  - gallamine
  - metocurine
  - pancuronium
  - pipecuronium
  - tubocurine
  - vecuronium
- Effectiveness decreased with
  - calcium
  - vitamin D
- Alters blood level of (increases or decreases) lithium
- Decreases metabolism and increases toxicity risk
  - carbamazipine
  - cyclosporine

- Procainamide
- Propranolol
- Quinidine gluconate
- Sodium bicarbonate
- Sodium nitroprusside

Incompatibilities
- Albumin

    – prazosin
    – quinidine
- Increased anesthetic effect
    – etodinate
- May produce severe hypotension
    – fentanyl
- Increases risk of toxicity
    – theophyllin

XYLOCAINE HCL (LIDOCAINE)

Classification: Antiarrhythmic (Class Ib)

Indications
Ventricular dysrhythmias including VT, VF, and digitalis-induced ventricular ectopy. Therapeutic effect: control of ventricular dysrhythmias

Contraindications
Hypersensitivity to amine local anesthetics, Stokes–Adams disease, complete heart block, second- or third-degree heart block, sinus bradycardia. **Note:** Use cautiously in CHF, respiratory depression, shock, heart block, elderly and patients <50 kg in weight, pregnancy, or lactation

Preparation/Administration
- IV bolus: 50–100 mg or 1.0–1.5 mg/kg
  - may repeat in 5–10 min
  - follow with continuous infusion of 1–4 mg/min
  - maximum dose: 3 mg/kg

Monitor the therapeutic drug level, which should be in the 1.2–5.0 µg/mL range.

Compatibilities
- D$_5$W
- D$_5$ lactated Ringer's
- Lactated Ringer's
- NaCl 0.45%
     0.9%
- Alteplase
- Aminophyllin
- Amrinone (INOCOR)
- Bretylium
- Calcium salts
- Cimetidine
- Dexamethasone
- Digoxin
- Dobutamine
- Dopamine
- Heparin

- Lasix
- Solu-Cortef
- Nitroglycerin
- Phenylephrine
- Potassium chloride
- Procainamide
- Sodium bicarbonate
- Verapamil

Adverse Effects
- Respiratory depression or arrest
- Seizure
- Loss of consciousness
- Hypotension
- Bradycardia
- Cardiovascular collapse

Drug Interactions
- Cimetidine or propanolol may result in increased serum concentrations of lidocaine resulting in toxicity

Dosage/Flow-Rate Chart
Dilution/Concentration[†]

Dosage (mcg/min)	mL/hr or microdrops/min
1	15
2	30
3	45
4	60

[†]1 g/250 mL (4 mg/mL). To infuse in milliliters/hr or microdrops/min.

The most effective and least complicated method of administering IV drugs is with tubing that delivers 60 gtts/cc.

BIBLIOGRAPHY

Abbokinase® urokinase for injection (February 1992), Abbott Laboratories (One Abbott Park Rd., Abbott Park, IL 60064-3500).

Activase® alteplase recombinant (January 1992, March 1995), Genentech, Inc. (460 Point San Bruno Boulevard, South San Francisco, CA 94080).

Activase® alteplase recombinant—*Pocket Reference Guide* (May 1992, March 1995), Genentech, Inc.

Adenocard IV (February 1992), Fujisawa Pharmaceutical Co. (3 Parkway North, Deerfield, IL 60015-2548).

Ahrens T, Rutherford K. The new pulmonary math applying the a/A ratio. *Am J Nurs* 87:337A–340H, 1987.

Algona P. Synergyst™ II—Clinical investigation underway. Minneapolis: *Medtronic News*, 1988.

American Heart Association. *Textbook of advanced cardiac life support.* Dallas: American Heart Association, 1987.

American Medical Association. *Guidelines for cardiopulmonary resuscitation and emergency cardiac care—JAMA.* Chicago: American Medical Association, 1992.

Aminosyn RF 5% (January 1987), Abbott Laboratories.

Aminophyllin injection (June 1990), Abbott Laboratories.

Andreoli K, Zipes D, Wallace A, Kinney M, Fowkes V (Eds.). *Comprehensive cardiac care,* 6th ed. St. Louis: Mosby, 1987.

Ayers S, Gregory J, Buehler M. *Cardiology: a clinicophysiological approach.* New York: Appleton-Century Crofts, 1971.

Bean D. *Introduction to ECG interpretation.* Rockville, MD: Aspen Publishers, 1987.

BEAR® 1000 ventilator—Training aid (September 1994), BEAR Medical Systems, Inc. (2085 Rustin Ave., Riverside, CA 92507-2460).

Berk J, Sampliner J (Eds.). *Handbook of critical care,* 3rd ed. Boston: Little, Brown, 1990.

Birdsall C. Hemofiltration, when? why? how? *Am J Nurs* 85:646, 1985

Blakemore esophageal nasogastric tube (1985). Davol Inc. (100 Sockanossett Crossroad, Cranston, RI 02920).

Brannon P, Tower S. Ventricular failure: New therapy using the mechanical assist device. *Crit Care Nurs* 6:70–85, 1986.

Braunwald E. *Heart disease—A textbook of cardiovascular medicine,* Vol. 1. Philadelphia: Saunders, 1984.

Braunwald E. *Heart disease—A textbook of cardiovascular medicine,* Vol. 2. Philadelphia: Saunders, 1984.

Brevibloc® injection (September 1993)—Dosage card (1995). Ohmeda Inc. (110 Allen Road, PO Box 804, Liberty Corner, NJ 97938-0804).

Bretylol® injection (January 1991), DuPont Pharmaceuticals (PO Box 363, Manati, Puerto Rico 00701).

Budassi SA, Barber J. *Mosby's manual of emergency care,* 2nd ed. St. Louis: Mosby, 1984.

Butler S. Current trends in autologous transfusion. *Reg Nurs* 52:44–55, 1989.

Camp L. Care of the groshong catheter. *Oncol Nurs Forum* 15:745–749, 1988.

Campbell J, Frisse M (Eds.). *Manual of medical therapies,* 24th ed. Boston: Little, Brown, 1983.

Capoten® tablets (July 1992), ER Squibb & Sons, Inc. (PO Box 4500, Princeton, NJ 08543-4500).

Cardiac auscultation—Study guide. St. Paul: 3M Health Care Group, 1987.

Cardiac pacing and patient care. Minneapolis: Medtronic Inc., 1987.

Cardizem® dosing card—DP #1171–9414700CVM (September 1993), Marion Merrell Dow Inc. (9300 Ward Parkway, Kansas City, MO 64114-0480).

Cardizem® injectable (October 1991, November 1992), Marion Merrell Dow Inc.

Case studies in intra-aortic balloon pumping. Clinical Educational Services, Paramus, NJ: Datascope Corp., 1989.

Central venous catheter care (January 1989), Quinton Instrument Co. (2121 Terry Avenue, Seattle, Washington 98121-2791).

Chad Therapeutics. *Oxymizer—oxygen conserving devices* (9445 De Soto Ave., Chatsworth, CA 91311), 1995.

Condon R, Nyhus L (Eds.). *Manual of surgical therapeutics,* 5th ed. Boston: Little, Brown, 1981.

Conover MB. *Understanding electrocardiography: Arrhythmias and the 12-lead EKG,* 5th ed. St. Louis: Mosby, 1988.

Continuous Cardiac Output and Mixed Venous Oxygen Saturation Monitoring System: CCOmbo™ and CCOmbo™ VIP™ Catheter and Vigilance® Monitor. Baxter Healthcare Corporation (PO Box 1150, Santa Ana, CA 92711), 1995.

Continuous Cardiac Output Monitoring System: IntelliCath™

and Vigilance®. Baxter Healthcare Corporation (Santa Ana, CA), 1995.

Cooney M, Perrone M. *Nurse review—A clinical update system,* Vol. 1: *Cardiac problems—cardiac arrest/cardiac trauma; dysrhythmias.* Springhouse, PA: Springhouse Corp., Nursing '87 Books, 1987.

Cordarone® intravenous-amiodarone hydrochloride (1995), Wyeth Laboratories, Inc. (PO Box 8922, Philadelphia, PA 19101).

Cordarone® tablets (October 1990), Wyeth Laboratories, Inc.

Crabble R. *Nurse review—A clinical update system,* Vol. 1: *Neurological problems—ICP monitoring; special neurological problems.* Springhouse Corp., Nursing '87 Books, 1987.

Crawford MV, Spence MI. *Commonsense approach to coronary care,* 6th ed. St. Louis, Mosby-Year Book, Inc., 1995.

Crisis drugs—clinical skillbuilders. Springhouse Corp., 1991.

CritiCath™ four-lumen catheter/PentaCath™ five-lumen thermodilution catheter (1988), Viggo-Spectramed (1900 Williams Drive, Oxnard, CA 93030).

Critical care in the 90s. Innovative Healthcare Inc. Minneapolis, MN: Genentech Inc., 1995.

Crockett P, Droppert B, Higgins S. *Defibrillation: What you should know.* Redmond, WA: Physio-Control, 1991.

Crockett P, McHugh L. *Noninvasive pacing: What you should know.* Redmond, WA: Physio-Control, 1988.

Damsgard C. *Nurse review—A clinical update system,* Vol. 1: *Gastrointestinal problems—Upper GI disorders.* Springhouse Corp., Nursing '87 Books, 1987.

Deglin J, Vallerand A. *Davis's drug guide for nurses,* 3rd ed. Philadelphia: Davis, 1993.

DeGroot K, Damato M (Eds.). *Critical care skills.* Los Altos, CA: Appleton & Lange, 1987.

Dente A, Lester R. *Intravenous medications for critical care.* Philadelphia: Saunders, 1989.

Dextrose injections (October 1988), Baxter Healthcare Corp. (1425 Lake Cook Rd., Deerfield, IL 60015).

Dextrose injections, 20%–70% (August 1988), Abbott Laboratories.

Dextrose 5% and Ringer's injection, dextrose 5% and LR injections (October 1984), Abbott Laboratories.

Dextrose and sodium chloride injections (July 1985), Abbott Laboratories.

Dilantin—phenytoin sodium injection (July 1993). Park-Davis (201 Tabor Rd., Morris Plains, NJ 07950).

Dillon D. Understanding mechanical ventilation. *Crit Care Nurs* 8:42–54, 1988.

Doering K. *Nurse review—A clinical update system,* Vol. 1: *Gastrointestinal problems—Lower GI.* Springhouse Corp., Nursing '87 Books, 1987.

Doyle E. *Nurse review—A clinical update system,* Vol. 1: *Gastrointestinal problems—GI emergencies.* Springhouse Corp., Nursing '87 Books, 1987.

Drug facts and comparisons. Philadelphia: Lippincott, 1988.

Du Pen® long-term epidural catheter—Use and maintenance. Cranston, RI: Davol Inc., 1979.

Elsenhans V. *Nurse review—A clinical update system,* Vol. 1: *Genitourinal problems—Urinary tract obstruction.* Springhouse Corp., Nursing '87 Books, 1987.

Emanuelsen K, Rosenlicht J (Eds.). *Handbook of critical care.* New York: John Wiley & Sons, 1986.

Emergency drug compatibility. Westborough, MA: Astra Pharmaceutical Products, Inc. (50 Otis St., Westboro, MA 01581-4500), 1987.

Eminase® anistreplase (April 1991), SmithKline Beecham Pharmaceuticals (One Franklin Plaza, PO Box 7929, Philadelphia, PA 19101).

Eminase® anistreplase—Handbook (January 1990), SmithKline Beecham Pharmaceuticals.

Epinephrine injection—1:1000 (July 1993). Elkins-Sinn, Inc. (2 Esterbrook Lane, Cherry Hill, NJ 08003-4099).

Erickson B. *Heart sounds: Adult cardiac abnormalities.* New Orleans: National Teaching Institute, 1987.

Ervin G. *Memory bank for critical care—EKGs and cardiac drugs,* 3rd ed. Baltimore: Williams & Wilkins, 1988.

Eubanks D, Bone R. *Comprehensive respiratory care.* St. Louis: Mosby, 1985.

Fearing M, Hart L. *Nurse review—A clinical update system,* Vol. 2: *Genitourinary problems—Acute and chronic renal failure.* Springhouse Corp., Nursing '87 Books, 1987.

Fre-Amine HBC 6.9% (June 1987), Kendall McGaw (2525 McGaw Avenue, Irvine, CA 92713).

Frye S, Lounsbury P. *Cardiac rhythm disorders—An introduction using the nursing process.* Baltimore: Williams & Wilkins, 1988.

Gahart B. *A handbook of intravenous medications,* 6th ed. St. Louis: Mosby, 1990.

Gallea B. The hemasite system: A transcutaneous approach to vascular access. *American Nephrology Nurses Association* 11:25–29, 60, 1984.

Goldschlager N, Goldman MJ. *Principles of clinical electrography,* 13th ed. Norwalk, CT: Appleton & Lange, 1989.

Gravenstein J, Paulus D, Hayes T. *Capnography in clinical practice.* Boston: Butterworths, 1989.

Green L. Nursing implications in the use of the multiple-lumen catheter. Santa Ana, CA: American Edwards Laboratories, 1986.

Halfman-Franey M. Current trends in hemodynamic monitoring of patients in shock. *Crit Care Nurs Q* 11:13–15, 1988.

Hardy S. SVO_2 continuous monitoring techniques. *Dimen Crit Care Nurs* 7:8–17, 1988.

Henry J. *Clinical diagnosis and management—By laboratory methods,* 17th ed. Philadelphia: Saunders, 1984.

Hensyl W, Felscher H, Cady B (Eds.). *Stedman's medical dictionary,* 25th ed. Baltimore: Williams & Wilkins, 1990.

Hudak C, Gallo B, Benz J. *Critical care nursing—A holistic approach,* 5th ed. Philadelphia: Lippincott, 1990.

Huestis D, Bove J, Busch S. *Practical blood transfusions,* 3rd ed. Boston: Little, Brown, 1981.

Hurst J, Logue R, Schlant R, Wenger N (Eds.). *The heart—Arteries and Veins,* 4th ed. New York: McGraw-Hill, 1979.

Hyperstat® IV injection (February 1985), Schering Corporation (2000 Galloping Hill Rd., Kenilworth, NJ 07033-0530).

Infuse-a-port implantable drug delivery system—Physician's manual. Norwood, MA: Shiley Infusaid Inc., 1987.

Inderal—propranolol hydrochloride (April 1992), Wyeth-Ayerst Co. (PO Box 8299, Philadelphia, PA 19101).

Inocor® lactate injection (November 1993), Sanofi Winthrop Pharmaceuticals (90 Park Avenue, New York, NY 10016).

Isordil—isosorbide dinitrate (October 1992). Wyeth-Ayerst Co.

Isuprel—isoproterenol hydrochloride injection (June 1993), Sanofi Winthrop Pharmaceuticals.

Johanson B, Wells S, Hoffmeister D, Dungca C. *Standards for critical care.* St. Louis: Mosby, 1988.

Kadas N. Reducing fluid overload with hemodialysis. *RN* 49:27–31, 1986.

Karb V, Queener S, Freeman J. *Handbook of drugs for nursing practice.* St. Louis: Mosby, 1989.

Kinney M, Dear C, Packa D, Voorman D (Eds.). *AACN's clinical reference for critical care nursing.* New York: McGraw-Hill, 1981.

Kopple J. *The renal patient—Profiles in nutritional management.* Chicago: Medical Directions, Inc., 1981.

Lanoxin® injection (September 1992). Burroughs Wellcome Co. (3030 Cornwallis Road, Research Triangle Park, NC 27709).

La Rocca J, Otto S. *Pocket guide to intravenous therapy.* St. Louis: Mosby, 1989.

Leahy N. *Quick reference to neurological critical care nursing.* Rockville, MD: Aspen Publishers, 1990.

Leslie D. *Nurse review—A clinical update system,* Vol. 1: *Neurological problems—Evaluation.* Springhouse Corp., Nursing '87 Books, 1987.

Levophed bitartrate (December 1991, April 1993), Sanofi Winthrop Pharmaceuticals.

LifePak 9P—Quik-Combo™ operating instructions, Physio-Control Corp. (Redmond, WA), January 1995.

Loebl S, Spratto G, Wit A. *The nurse's drug handbook.* New York: John Wiley & Sons, 1977.

Lonsway R. Care of the patient with an epidural catheter. *J Intraven Nurs* 11:52–55, 1988.

Ludmer P, Goldschlager N. Cardiac pacing in the 80s. *N Engl J Med* 311:1671–1680, 1984.

Managing IV therapy—Nursing Books '82. Springhouse, PA: Springhouse Corp., 1982.

Marini J, Wheeler A. Critical care medicine—The essentials. Baltimore: Williams & Wilkins, 1989.

Marriott H. Practical electrocardiography, 8th ed. Baltimore: Williams & Wilkins, 1988.

Marriott H, Conover M. Advanced concepts in arrhythmias, 2nd ed. St. Louis: Mosby, 1989.

McEvoy G, Litvak K, McQuarrie G, Schmadel L (Eds.). AHFS drug information. Bethesda, MD: American Society of Hospital Pharmacists, 1990.

McEvoy G, Litvak D, Welsh O, Douglas P, Kester L (Eds.). AHFS drug information. Bethesda, MD: American Society of Hospital Pharmacists, 1993.

McSwain N. Pneumatic anti-shock garment: State of the art. Am Emerg Med 17:506–525, 1988.

Means B, Taplett L. Quick reference to critical care. Rockville, MD: Aspen Publishers, 1988.

Medical anti-shock trousers (1988), David Clark Co. (360 Franklin Street, Box 15054, Worcester, MA 01615-0054).

Meter M. Clinical facts and formulas—A pocket guide. Maple Glen, PA: Marvan, 1987.

Millar S, Sampson L, Soukup S. AACN procedure manual for critical care, 2nd ed. Philadelphia: Saunders, 1985.

Miracle V. Anatomy of a murmur. Nursing '86 17:26–31, 1986.

Moghissi K, Boore J. Parenteral and enteral nutrition for nurses. Rockville, MD: Aspen Publishers, 1983.

Mohsen Z, Janeway C, Cooke R. Pediatrics. Boston: Little, Brown, 1975.

Monitoring fluids and electrolytes precisely—Nursing '78. Horsham, PA: Intermed Communications, 1978.

Moses H, Taylor G, Schneider J, Dover J. A practical guide to cardiac pacing, 2nd ed. Boston: Little, Brown, 1987.

National Heart, Lung and Blood Institute. Blood disease and resources (7550 Wisconsin Ave., Bethesda, MD 20892).

Nentwich P. Handbook of intravenous medications. Boston: Jones and Bartlett Publishers, 1991.

Neo-synephrine® hydrochloride (July 1992), Sanofi Winthrop Pharmaceuticals.

Nikas D (Ed.). The critically ill neurosurgical patient. New York: Churchill Livingston, 1982.

Nitropress® (December 1990), Abbott Laboratories.

Norcuron—vecuronium bromide—for injection (January 1992), Organon Inc. (375 Mount Pleasant Ave., West Orange, NJ 07052).

Nursing Photobook™—Providing respiratory care, Nursing '82 Books. Horsham, PA: Intermed Communications, Inc., 1982.

Nursing Photobook™—Using monitors, Nursing '81 Books. Horsham, PA: Intermed Communications, Inc., 1981.

Nursing '90 IV drug handbook. Springhouse, PA: Springhouse Corp., 1990.

Orland M, Saltman R (Eds.). Manual of medical therapeutics, 25th ed. Boston: Little, Brown, 1986.

Pacemaker code and rate and interval conversion—Pocket reference (April 1995), Minneapolis: Medtronic Inc.

Pancoast P (Ed.). Drug formulary—for MHG. Hudson, OH: Lexi-Comp Inc., 1992.

Papper S, Coussons T, Williams G (Eds.). Manual of medical

care of the surgical patient, 3rd ed. Boston: Little, Brown, 1981.

Pechan M. *Coronary care modules.* Baltimore: Williams & Wilkins, 1987.

Perry B. Our experience with the Port-a-Cath™ system. *Alberta Assoc Reg Nurs* 44:25–27, 1988.

Peterson K, Brown M. Extracorporeal membrane oxygenation in adults: A Nursing challenge. *Focus Crit Care* 17:40–49, 1990.

Phillips R, Feeney M. *The cardiac rhythms—A systematic approach to interpretation,* 2nd ed. Philadelphia: Saunders, 1980.

Pittiglio D, Baldwin A, Sohmer P (Eds.). *Modern blood banking and transfusion practices.* Philadelphia: Davis, 1983.

Plan of care for the patient/family requiring intra-aortic balloon pump therapy—In a nursing diagnosis framework. Clinical Education Services, Paramus, NJ: Datascope Corp., 1988.

Potassium chloride for injection concentration, USP (April 1992), Abbott Laboratories.

Primacor® IV (November 1994), Sanofi Winthrop Pharmaceuticals.

ProcalAmine—3% amino acid and 3% glycerin injection with electrolytes (September 1989), Kendall McGaw.

Professional guide to diseases, 3rd ed. Springhouse, PA: Springhouse Corp., 1989.

Purcell J, Burrows S. A pacemaker primer. *Am J Nurs* 85:553–568, 1985.

Purcell J, Pippin L, Mitchell M. Intra-aortic balloon pump therapy. *Am J Nurs* 83:775–779, 1983.

Renaflo® II hemofiltration system, Renal Systems (14605 28th Avenue North, Minneapolis, MN 55447), May 1993.

Rich M. *Coronary care for the house officer.* Baltimore: Williams & Wilkins, 1989.

Riley J. Intracranial pressure monitoring made easy. *RN* 44:53–57, 1981.

Ringer's injection (February 1984), Travenol (1425 Lake Cook Rd., Deerfield, IL 60015).

Riser S. Patient care manual for implanted vascular access devices. *J Intraven Nurs* 11:166–168, 1988.

Rosen H, Calic M. An epidural analgesia program: Balancing risks and benefits. *Crit Care Nurs* 10:32–41, 1990.

Ross A. *Nurse review—A clinical update system,* Vol. 1: *Neurological problems—Nontraumatic disorders.* Springhouse Corp., Nursing '87 Books, 1987.

Rotating tourniquets—Procedure manual. Gulfport, MS: Memorial Hospital at Gulfport, 1989.

Roth L. *Mosby's drug reference.* St. Louis: Mosby, 1989.

Satinder JS, Goldschlager N. Selecting the best cardiac pacing system. *Choic Cardiol* 3:22–26, 1989.

Schnittger I. The role of AV conduction in the selection of an optimal pacing mode. Minneapolis: *Medtronic News,* 1988.

Schroeder C. Pulse oximetry: A nursing care plan. *Crit Care Nurs* 8:50–66, 1988.

Sectral—acebutolol hydrochloride (August 1992). Wyeth Laboratories Inc.

Seminar for intra-aortic balloon pumping. Clinical Education Services, Paramus, NJ: Datascope Corp., 1986.

Sheehy S, Baker J. *Emergency nursing principles and practices,* 2nd ed. St. Louis: Mosby, 1985.

Sheehy S, Marvin J, Jimmerson C. *Manual of clinical trauma care—The first hour.* St. Louis: Mosby, 1989.

Shoemaker W, Thompson W, Holbrook P. *Textbook of critical care.* Philadelphia: Saunders, 1984.

Sibbald W. *Synopsis of critical care,* 3rd ed. Baltimore: Williams & Wilkins, 1988.

Sifton D, Westley G, Pfohl B (Eds.). *Physicians' desk reference,* 48th ed. Montvale, NJ: Medical Economics Data Production Co., 1994.

Silber E, Katz L. *Heart disease.* New York: Macmillan, 1975.

Sodium bicarbonate injection, USP (September 1993), Abbott Laboratories.

Sodium chloride injections (October 1988), Abbott Laboratories.

Sokolow M, McIlroy M. *Clinical cardiology,* 2nd ed. Los Altos, CA: Lange Medical Publishers, 1979.

Stillwell S. *Mosby's critical care nursing reference.* St. Louis: Mosby Year Book, 1992.

Streptase—streptokinase (December 1987), Hoechst-Roussel Pharmaceuticals Inc. (PO Box 2500, Somerville, NJ 00876-1258).

Swan-Ganz® pacing-TD catheters (1988), Baxter Healthcare Corp.

Swearingen P, Keen J. *Manual of critical care—Applying nursing diagnosis to adult critical illness,* 2nd ed. St. Louis: Mosby Year Book, 1991.

Swearingen P, Sommers M, Miller K. *Manual of critical care—Applying nursing diagnosis.* St. Louis: Mosby, 1988.

Sweetwood H. *Clinical electrocardiogram for nurses,* 2nd ed. Rockville, MD: Aspen Publishing, 1989.

Synder E, Kennedy M (Eds.). *Blood transfusion therapy—A physician's handbook.* Arlington, VA: American Association of Blood Banks, 1983.

Talbot L, Marquardt M. *Pocket guide to critical care assessment.* St. Louis: Mosby, 1989.

Tambocor—flecainide acetate (June 1992). 3M Pharmaceuticals (PO Box 33275, St. Paul, MN 55144-1000).

Taylor J. *Nurse review—A clinical update system,* Vol. 1: *Respiratory problems—Airway obstruction.* Springhouse Corp., Nursing '87 Books, 1987.

Temporary pacemaker code and rate and interval conversion—Pocket reference (1992), Medtronic.

Tennant D, Stone K. Skills competency testing for the Thoraklex® chest drainage system and cardiovascular autotransfusion unit (February 1995). Cranston, RI: Davol, Inc.

The future of SVO$_2$ monitoring (1988). Oxnard, CA: Viggo-Spectramed.

Thelan L, Davie J, Urden L, Kritek P. *Textbook of critical care diagnosis and management.* St. Louis: Mosby, 1990.

Thompson J, McFarland G, Hirsch J, Tucker S, Bowers A. *Clinical nursing.* St. Louis: Mosby, 1986.

Tilkian A, Daily E. *Cardiovascular procedures.* St. Louis: Mosby, 1986.

Tressel L. *Handbook of injectable drugs.* Bethesda, MD: American Society of Hospital Pharmacists, 1993.

Underhill S, Woods S, Froelisher E, Halpenny C. *Cardiac nursing,* 2nd ed. Philadelphia: Lippincott, 1989.

Understanding hemodynamic measurements made with the Swan-Ganz® catheter. Santa Ana, CA: American Edwards Laboratories, 1987.

Update on temporary and permanent pacemaker use, Medtronic Inc., 1990.

Valle G, Lemberg L. Effective technique of controlling volume in refractory congestive heart failure. *Heart Lung* 16:712–717, 1987.

VanRiper S, VanRiper J. *Nurse review—A clinical update sys-*

tem, Vol. 1: *Cardiac problems—Myocardial infarction.* Springhouse Corp., Nursing '87 Books, 1987.

Viall C. Your complete guide to central venous catheters. *Nurs '90* 20:34–41, 1990.

Wallace L, Wardell S. *Nursing pharmacology—A comprehensive approach to drug therapy,* 2nd ed. Boston: Jones and Bartlett Publishers, 1992.

Walsh S, Bank L. How to insert a small-bore feeding tube safely. *Nurs '90* 20:55–61, 1990.

Wesley J, Khalidi N, Faubian W, Baker W, Lott B, Hickisch S, Coran A (Eds.). *The University of Michigan hospital parenteral and enteral nutritional manual,* 2nd ed. Chicago: Abbott Laboratories, 1982.

White K. Completing the hemodynamic picture: SVO_2. *Heart Lung* 14:272–279, 1989.

Whitney R. Hickman, Groshong and venous access ports: Can you tell the difference? New Orleans: The National AJN Conference on Medical-Surgical and Geriatric Nursing, 1990.

Widman F (Ed.). *American Association of Blood Banks— Technical manual,* 9th ed. Arlington, VA: American Association of Blood Banks, 1985.

Wilson R (Ed.). *Principles and techniques of critical care.* Kalamazoo, MI: Upjohn Co., 1976.

Winters V. Implantable vascular access devices. *Oncol Nurs Forum* 1:25–30, 1984.

Woodley M, Whelan A (Eds.). *Manual of medical therapeutics,* 27th ed. Boston: Little, Brown, 1992.

Wright J, Shelton B. *Desk reference for critical care nursing.* Boston: Jones and Bartlett Publishers, 1993.

Zeller F, Anders R. Compatibility of intravenous drugs on a coronary intensive care unit. *Drug Intell Clin Pharm* 20: 349–352.

Zozier B, Erb G. *Techniques in clinical nursing.* Redwood City, CA: Addison-Wesley, 1989.

Zygmont D. *Nurse review—A clinical update system,* Vol. 1: *Respiratory problems—Evaluating common oxygen delivery systems; intrinsic lung disease.* Springhouse Corp., Nursing '87 Books, 1987.

CPSIA information can be obtained
at www.ICGtesting.com
Printed in the USA
LVHW050933010223
738389LV00028B/169